Clinical Management of Feeding Disorders: Case Studies

TWO ENDORSEMENTS OF THE YOSSEM METHOD OF FEEDING THERAPY FROM A CAREGIVER AND A PATIENT

I remember leaving that first therapy session with the feeling that there was so much work ahead of us. Michelle's handicaps were severe, and both my husband and I felt that eating was not only a necessity, but also an important pleasure that we didn't want Michelle to be without. Meals were a family time in which we wanted Michelle to participate as more than just an observer.

Various feeding therapists had suggested a feeding tube for Michelle, telling us that she would never be able to chew or swallow well. This would never have been acceptable to us, but may have been a necessity, had we not been fortunate enough to be recommended to Florence Yossem.

There was a great deal of work ahead: immediate changes in positioning, food consistency, spoon placement, exercises designed to aid lip closure, drinking from a cup. Florence's ideas and methods were very different from those of other feeding experts. But Florence was also different from other experts.

Florence created a therapy atmosphere in which I believed I would be able to succeed in teaching Michelle new skills. I felt that Florence was just as invested in our success as I was. Michelle was not a case, she was a person. I left each session with motivation to continue, even when some weeks brought little progress.

What Florence knew that I didn't was that the new skills we learned from her would make Michelle more of a real member of the family. Eventually, my husband as well as our other children were able to feed Michelle. This brought Michelle closer to all of us and all of us closer to each other. Such success must be what motivates this very special lady.

Mother of Michelle (The Case of Many Challenges)

My strange and inexplicable difficulties with swallowing had turned one of the most essential and potentially pleasurable of human experiences—eating—into a dreadful experience. I was near the end of my rope, after seeking help for several years from a variety of physicians and other health-care specialists, none of whom had ever heard of a problem like mine and were quite unable to help me. In fact, I had virtually given up on ever being able to eat normally again, when a friend recommended Florence Yossem. "She's a terrific feeding therapist," my friend told me. I had never even *heard* of feeding therapy! In my first visit with Ms. Yossem, I could clearly see that she was quite experienced in such matters and—unlike the other health-care professionals I had consulted—did not seem the least bit surprised when I described my problems to her. She immediately put me at ease and, after observing my swallowing habits closely and studying my videofluoroscopy, she came up with a regimen of exercises for me. At each session, she was extremely attentive and obviously understood the nature of the mechanical problems I was suffering. She never made me feel pressured and was always able to tailor her "homework" assignments to be as constructive as possible. Though these assignments were sometimes tedious and challenging, they were well-designed to fit my own abilities at any given time and were never unreasonably difficult. They definitely led me to a slow and steady improvement, and my years of frustration finally came to an end.

Only those who have experienced difficulties with swallowing can imagine the everyday frustration (not to mention the hunger!) that such problems can cause. The ability to overcome these problems has led to a radical improvement in my life, for the capacity to nourish and enjoy myself and interact socially with others is absolutely crucial. Ms. Yossem is truly a talented healer, and her positive effect on my own everyday life has been incalculable.

Dorothy (The Case of the University Professor)

Clinical Management of Feeding Disorders: Case Studies

Florence L. Yossem, M.A., O.T.R.
Eugene, Oregon

With a foreword by
Doris M. Okada, Ph.D.
Professor of Special Education and
Director, Infant-Toddler Development Center,
California State University, Dominguez Hills

Illustrations by
Kate Pryka

Butterworth–Heinemann
Boston Oxford Johannesburg Melbourne New Delhi Singapore

Butterworth–Heinemann supports the efforts of American Forests and the Global ReLeaf program in its campaign for the betterment of trees, forests, and our environment.

Library of Congress Cataloging-in-Publication Data
Yossem, Florence L.
    Clinical management of feeding disorders: case studies / Florence
L. Yossem ; with a foreword by Doris M. Okada.
        p.   cm.
    Includes bibliographical references and index.
    ISBN 0-7506-9854-3
    1. Deglutition disorders--Case studies. I. Title.
    [DNLM: 1. Deglutition Disorders--therapy.   2. Feeding Behavior.
WI 250 Y65c 1997]
RC815.2.Y67 1997
616.3'106--dc21
DNLM/DLC
for Library of Congress   97-27402
                                                                      CIP

British Library Cataloguing-in-Publication Data
A catalogue record for this book is available from the British Library.

Contents

Foreword

I first met Florence Yossem in the early 1970s, a time of de-institutionalization and the initiation of public school programs for individuals with profound developmental disabilities in California, as she was developing and implementing feeding programs for this population. With a dearth of information in the field, there was a tremendous need for therapeutic interventions, especially with children. These pioneering efforts evolved into the Yossem Method.

In subsequent years, Ms. Yossem served as a feeding therapy consultant for our on-campus early intervention program; offered college classes and workshops for special educators, occupational therapists, speech-language pathologists, and other professionals; and worked with children and their parents and adults in their homes. As her work and training programs expanded beyond California to the other western states, Ms. Yossem also increased her repertoire of cases.

This book presents, through challenging and at times formidable case studies, the essential components of the Yossem Method: thorough assessment, analysis, strategies, and evaluation. Melding theory with successful practice, the book is based on the author's rich and varied experiences and many years of refining her methodology.

Special educators, occupational therapists, speech-language pathologists, and other professionals who work with individuals with feeding needs in a variety of settings will find a wealth of information in this book. My former students who were trained by Ms. Yossem attest to the effectiveness of her method in dealing with a range of problems from positioning to swallowing to feeding as they teach each day in their special education classrooms.

Doris M. Okada, Ph.D.

Preface

Few problems in life require more care and patience than feeding and swallowing dysfunctions. In response to numerous requests over the years by the colleagues, patients, and caregivers with whom I have been associated, I have undertaken the task of writing this book. I was specifically asked by all to write as I speak—in layperson's language. I sincerely hope that my efforts will stimulate interest and creativity in all who work in this field—that is, beginning and advanced occupational therapists, speech-language pathologists, physicians, physical therapists, nurses, nutritionists, family caregivers, special education teachers, principals and administrators, aides, and primary health care providers.

This book is divided in sections to help guide the reader into my world of functional therapy management. Part I offers information and background. Parts II and III offer case studies with specific, daily, individualized treatment techniques. Patient ages range from the very young to the elderly. Some of the patients were seen privately, others in school settings, residential facilities, and consultation situations. Part IV details the how, why, and when of 17 treatment techniques—with illustrations.

Many years have passed since I began my work. I sincerely hope that this book will be of value. I am forever grateful to all of my patients and caregivers who have not only included me as a part of their families, but who also have taught me treatment management.

Florence L. Yossem

Acknowledgments

This book has been long in coming, and it is to the credit of many colleagues, patients, caregivers, and friends that it has finally arrived.

My deepest gratitude and heartfelt thanks, however, go to my remarkable daughter Deborah S. Kelly, without whom this book would never have been written. How she could transcribe my scribble to enter it into her computer, I'll never understand. Thank you, Deborah.

For encouragement and assistance, I especially thank my friend Marlene Mayers, a registered nurse and a fellow author, for her guidance and support throughout the writing of this book. I also thank Doris Okada, Ph.D., for her continuing support of my work over many years. Appreciation is also due to Melvin Cohen, Ph.D., who tried so hard, for so long, to encourage me to write this book.

I also extend gratitude to Diane Flores, Eunice Zee Chen, Nathalie Gittelman, Marcia Bates, and Herb Lieberman, who have guided, prodded, and worked with me to help produce this book. I also wish to thank my son-in-law, David Kelly, who provided important technical support and assistance.

To all of my patients and caregivers who have enriched my life by sharing theirs with me, I offer my enthusiastic "thank you" from the bottom of my heart.

Finally, but not least, I sincerely thank my editor, Karen Oberheim, for her kindness, support, competence, and patience.

Florence L. Yossem

I
Background

Introduction

Staring at the plant boxes filled with dazzling yellow flowers lined up against the windows of the first McDonald's restaurant to open in England, I never dreamed how much a part of my life that restaurant's hamburgers would become. Approximately 25 years have passed since that lovely day in London, but I remember it vividly even now. Working mainly with children, but also with patients of all ages who have an eating dysfunction, I have heard the same refrain hundreds of times: "When I am done with this therapy, I want to go to McDonald's." At that time, I had no idea that a desire for hamburgers would be a liturgy I would hear for the rest of my professional life!

Twenty-five years later, my opportunity to write has arrived. I am now eager to share my techniques with readers. As a registered occupational therapist with a master's degree in psychology, I have worked in a preschool nursery for children with disabilities; was a director of occupational therapy for children and adults at United Cerebral Palsy of Los Angeles, CA (a national network of local affiliates offering therapeutic programs and supportive services for persons with cerebral palsy and other developmental disabilities and their families); acted as a consultant to too many schools and adult day-care facilities to count; and taught my 2-day lecture and lab classes at hospitals and universities in various states and in Central America, Asia, and Canada. I have worked closely with parents and spouses, special educators, teachers, and aides, as well as with physicians, occupational therapists, physical therapists, speech and language therapists, nurses, nutritionists, school principals, and administrators of school districts for the developmentally disabled. My clinical practice has been most important to me, however, because it has provided intimate time with patients of all ages and their caregivers. All these years of clinical and practical experience have helped me to feel confident about determining the best treatment for each of my patients.

Because the manner in which I treated my patients worked effectively, I used the same functional approach in teaching my "student" colleagues. Functional treatment involves hands-on learning and practicing practical skill after practical skill. My lecture and lab courses focused on the same types of practical learning and were full of enthusiastic peers who expressed an eagerness to try the techniques presented while creatively thinking about new techniques.

Throughout the years, I have interacted with other specialists through consultation with physicians, therapists, and nutritionists in group meetings; informal conversations; and team projects frequently involving a physician, nurse, physical therapist, nutritionist, and the patient and spouse or the patient's parents. These interactions were directed at improving the quality of care for the patient by providing the service of a multidisciplinary team. My psychology degree has helped me to think across the disciplines, broadened my point of view, and enabled me to work more closely within family dynamics by creating a family-centered treatment plan.

The Yossem method of feeding therapy began to develop in 1968 when I met Helen Mueller, a speech pathologist from Switzerland who came to the University of California, Los Angeles, to discuss her theory of pre-speech feeding therapy. This therapy was based on the fact that the muscles for chewing and swallowing are the same muscles used for speech. Mueller was the first therapist to study the connection between pre-speech and feeding, and she began presenting her findings in Europe in 1963. The techniques she developed based on this connection seemed to be the answer for treating many of the feeding problems I had seen. At that time, a large number of my patients had severe cerebral palsy and would most likely never acquire clear or even adequate speech. However, Mueller's work helped me to see that pre-speech feeding therapy nonetheless had benefits for these patients because the oral-motor skills acquired could be used to aid in bilabial closure on a spoon, improved lip closure on a cup, improved tongue and jaw movements for chewing, and improved coordination of breathing and swallowing. I knew that I wanted to apply my energies and skills to this exciting new approach to treatment. Mueller's theories formed the basic foundation of a new avenue of treatment that I added to and subtracted from. My changes and modifications to her work were the basis for my own approach to dealing with patient problems in a physically and emotionally supportive environment.

When I first began my practice in 1965, published material on feeding therapy was not readily available. Therefore, Helen Mueller; Nancie R.F. Finnie, F.C.S.P.; and A. Jean Ayres, Ph.D., were the authors I turned to for information and ideas. I am deeply indebted to them for their research and writings. Numerous worthwhile books on developmental disabilities and feeding therapy have been written in the 1970s, 1980s, and 1990s by excellent clinicians. I list a number of them in the suggested reading list at the end of this book.

My treatment method focuses on function and attempts to encourage or restore "normal" responses to daily physical needs. Developing or restoring the skill of being able to eat well (and therefore safely) is my major goal in therapy. To accomplish that goal, I have always used hands-on techniques in working with the patient and caregiver. Therefore, I need to have a variety of functional treatment techniques in my repertoire. These techniques are explained in **Part IV**. The application of these techniques to specific cases is discussed in **Parts II and III**. These case studies demonstrate the importance of recognizing that *these techniques and exercises vary in their application, position, duration, and timing within the treatment plan.* The selected combination of these features makes each treatment plan individual. Just because the same techniques are being used to treat patients does not mean that the same treatment plan is being used.

In the case studies in **Parts II and III**, I do not discuss working with the "whole body" (except in reference to positioning and sensory defensiveness problems). The Yossem method does not emphasize working to normalize muscle tone of the whole body, but my results working with patients with disabilities and feeding problems were consistently successful. However, I always recommend other treatment modalities, such as occupational therapy, physical therapy, speech pathology, sensory integrative therapy, and nutrition therapy, to patients with inadequate muscle tone and abnormal reflexes and movement. New and improved methods of evaluation allow therapists to observe swallowing skills that cannot be seen in a "bedside" evaluation. This is seen in **The Case of the University Professor** (p. 41), in which we were able to use a modified barium-swallow videofluoroscopy. Although such new methods are vitally important, I also use my analytical background, my clinical experiences, my observations, and my intuition to guide my choice of treatment. Making use of all of these skills and experiences, I am able to maintain the ongoing connection necessary to improve the whole person.

The feeding problems of my patients have been due to a wide variety of conditions, including cerebral palsy, developmental disabilities and delay, degenerative disorders, mental retardation, Down syndrome, neurologic disorders, genetic dysfunction, dysautonomia, bronchial pulmonary dysphasia, failure to thrive, and numerous problems for which the diagnosis is not known. Specific manifestations of these conditions may include an open-mouth swallow, excessive drooling, rejection of certain food textures, inability to chew, inadequate tongue and jaw movements, pre-speech problems, tube feeding, slow swallows, loud swallows, slow eating, hypersensitivity and hyposensitivity to touch within the oral area, sensory defensiveness of the entire body, nasal regurgitation, vomiting, behavior problems, refusal to eat, frequent upper respiratory illnesses, coughing, and choking. Many patients with feeding disorders take medications to control seizures, which often makes treatment a challenge, as they may become sleepy, withdrawn, or overly excited. Some patients are referred by physicians and special education clinicians, but many are referred to my clinic by the families of my patients.

My approach to occupational therapy treatment deals only with the beginning stages of the swallow. These stages address muscle movements that improve lip closure, tongue movement, and jaw movements. Normal movements for drinking require bilabial closure on a cup. The tongue must form a groove to hold the liquid before the normal swallow occurs. The tongue must also move food within the mouth to form a bolus (see Glossary for definition). This bolus is then held between the tongue and the hard palate before swallowing. To chew normally, the jaw must move not only up and down but also in rotation. Nasal breathing and the swallow normally coordinate well so that the soft palate elevates and the patient breathes nasally until the swallow. Patients with feeding dysfunctions frequently have abnormal breathing and swallowing patterns. The swallow is initiated when the tongue begins to move the food or liquid backward.

Treating feeding dysfunction involves more than just treating oral problems. I am equally concerned about emotional and behavioral problems, as much as it is within my capabilities to address such problems. Patients of all ages with feeding disorders must deal with many emotions—denial, anger, guilt, hope, and depression—before they understand and accept what the future holds for them, which may include a lack of independence or the need to live in a special facility. They also must deal with confusion and fear of the unknown. In addition, there may be problems in the home and family due to the difficulty of dealing with the feeding disorder. Behavior problems may compound the ongoing stress of daily living. For parents of persons with disabilities, navigating treatments, special schools, and care facilities may be frightening. Therefore, I try to be available to support my patients and their families and caregivers. I listen and examine the problems they are facing and try to help resolve them without being intrusive. Establishing good rapport between the patient (and family) and the clinician is vital. I emphasize to the patient that we are *working together* as *we* write out the ongoing home program of therapeutic activities.

My work has always been my passion and I am eager to share my expertise with my readers. Working intimately with patients and their caregivers has been intensely rewarding as I watch their improvement and develop lasting relationships with them. Patients and caregivers work intensely over a period of months (or more), and I think they deserve an enormous amount of credit for their ability to work on overcoming their difficulties. I hope that this book will help readers understand why the Yossem method works and that it will open up clinical pathways that will be interesting, creative, and exciting.

In a few of the cases presented in **Parts II and III**, I have slightly simplified or abbreviated my discussion of the actual treatment process. Writing all of the details, difficulties, and discussions of each visit would be impossible. However, the treatment process, total amount of time involved, and conclusions are as accurate as possible. Not all diagnoses related to feeding disorders are discussed in the cases because I think that the techniques discussed here could serve as a basis for treatment of patients with many different diagnoses.

For the sake of clarity I use the term *patient* to identify all clients, private patients, students, residents, and others with whom I have worked. All names and identities have been changed to protect the persons involved.

Yossem Method of Feeding Therapy

PATIENT/THERAPIST RELATIONSHIP

When I first began working as a therapist, I thought I could help my patients in a simple, straightforward manner: evaluate the problem, establish a meaningful relationship with the patient and caregiver, set treatment goals, and designate exercises to be performed at home. It did not take long for me to recognize how many more things had to be considered. It has been my lifelong experience to have basically worked independently—in private practice; as a consultant working with children, adults, and staff; as a lecturer, teaching my techniques to my peers; and as a director of occupational therapy in a facility for adults with developmental disabilities. It is this background that has formed the manner in which I practice my skills, which my colleagues call the *Yossem method*.

Role of the Caregiver

Many of the patients I have treated depend on their caregivers to have most of their needs fulfilled. Feeding is, of course, one of the most important of those needs. Therefore, in my practice, the *caregiver is as important as the patient*. In the Yossem method, the parent, teacher, aide, spouse, therapist, or nurse actually performs the hands-on treatment with the patient. The required daily treatment is lengthy, time consuming, and frustrating. The patient and caregiver need to be considerate of each other, flexible, caring, and patient. Because the Yossem method requires the therapist to work through the caregiver, it is essential that the therapist fully understand the relationship between the caregiver, the patient, and himself or herself. The ability of all three treatment participants to understand the others' emotions, needs, and concerns is an important determinant of therapy outcome. **The Case of the Mysterious Ailment** (p. 65) demonstrates this need. In this particular case, I came to understand the need of the patient's mother for control and quick treatment results. When I understood this, I was able to help her see and feel her son's need to move more slowly and determine his rate of progression.

Comfort Zone

Many of my patients and their caregivers have been to numerous therapists and clinics before coming to me. Therefore, I believe that it is important to explore the caregiver's and patient's readiness to accept new avenues of thought and treatment techniques without feeling that they are giving up control over treatment. All caregivers and patients need to express their fears, frustrations, and needs on an ongoing basis. Understanding these fears and expectations is part of understanding the comfort zones of the patient and caregiver. This comfort zone reflects the trust and confidence the patient and caregiver place in the therapist and their willingness to try new treatments. The therapist must maintain this confidence by being honest and straightforward about changes, reasonable expectations, disappointments, and progress. Therapy may last for 1 year or longer, making the development of patient and caregiver confidence in the therapist an ongoing process.

DIAGNOSTIC PROCESS

Initial Evaluation

During the initial visit with the primary caregiver and patient, information, including medical history and medications, past and present feeding problems, and oral intake, should be gathered. The specific components of a complete oral-motor feeding evaluation are outlined on p. 15. I have found it best to devote two sessions to this evaluation so that the patient and caregiver feel that the evaluation is proceeding at a relaxed pace. This two-session evaluation allows me to make closer observations and establish rapport with the patient and caregiver. Oral-motor dysfunction and feeding problems are frequently only one part of a total problem; therefore, the *whole person* needs to be observed. Posture, positioning, ambulation, breathing and swallowing patterns, reflex patterns, motor control, communication ability, developmental level, and sensory deprivation (i.e., rejection of touch) should all be noted during the evaluation. By encouraging conversation throughout the evaluation, I begin to develop a relationship with the patient and caregiver and also gain information about the patient's awareness of his or her surroundings and situation, comprehension, communication skills, prespeech needs, and desire to cooperate.

Because patients with feeding disorders often are unable (or too young) to effectively express their concerns through verbal communication, observation is of paramount importance in the evaluation. Also, I try to listen carefully "between the lines" to discover unspoken problems or misconceptions. These patients need to be understood! This may be especially effective in learning more about the caregiver's concerns. Comments such as "Billy doesn't talk or make many sounds," "Oh Mary, she's just lazy (or stubborn)," or "Johnny has a cold and that's why he can't close his lips on the spoon" all may provide information about the source of the feeding disorder and its concomitant problems. These comments by caregivers provide an excellent opportunity for the therapist to educate the caregiver (and patient, if appropriate) about the nature of feeding disorders. I often review the basic developmental steps required for the patient to close his or her lips on a spoon, chew, drink from a cup, and speak. I also explain that the speech and chewing muscles are the same, and that problems in these areas are often interrelated. However, I am careful to stress that speech may *not* occur even with successful feeding therapy. Caregivers frequently are unaware or in denial of a problem. Educating the patient and caregiver helps develop their confidence in the therapeutic process.

Feeding Evaluation

I complete a feeding evaluation during the initial visit with a patient. The patient or caregiver brings favorite foods in snack form, and I add additional foods so that the variety of textures needed to complete a full observation of oral-motor skills is available. This evaluation is best done at the most opportune feeding time for the patient (the time the patient usually eats a meal). I first ask the caregiver to feed the patient (or have the patient eat independently), so that I may observe feeding techniques and problems. Following this, I feed the patient. My primary concerns are preventing aspiration, providing adequate nutrition, and determining future treatment needs. This *hands-on evaluation is repeated throughout the patient's treatment* in order to set treatment priorities.

Videofluoroscopy

Videofluoroscopy (the modified barium swallow) may be recommended, particularly if aspiration is a concern. "Silent" aspiration (when the patient neither coughs nor chokes) is often overlooked in initial evaluations. It is vital that any aspiration be noted and the patient thoroughly examined. Before videofluoroscopy was available, many of my patients were, of necessity, assessed by what is called the "bedside" evaluation. Today, we have access to radiologic techniques to diagnose aspiration and other unseen problems.

TREATMENT

The Yossem method of feeding therapy is centered around a home-based program of exercises performed at least three times daily. The overall success of treatment depends on the success of the home program and, therefore, on patient and caregiver understanding of the home program and agreement and compliance with it. Because the caregiver and patient will be responsible for the success of this home program, I make sure they are comfortable with all parts of the treatment plan. I do not outline a treatment plan and then present it to the patient and caregiver; instead, the three of us work as a team to set goals and then develop an appropriate home program. Teachers and residential facility caregivers also have prescribed time segments and facility regulations to follow, and therefore must work therapy into gross or fine motor skills time periods, snack periods, or meal times.

I consider the patient, caregiver, and myself to be the primary treatment team. This primary treatment team is supported by a larger multidisciplinary team made up of physicians, educational specialists, occupational therapists, physical therapists, speech-language pathologists, nurses, nutritionists, teachers, and aides. One or more of these persons may be consulted frequently.

Goals

The first step in outlining a treatment plan is setting goals. Long-term goals for feeding-disorder therapy frequently include one or more of the following: improving positioning; improving oral intake and nutrition; transitioning from pureed or strained foods to textured foods; and developing chewing skills and normal breathing and swallowing patterns. I break long-term goals down into short-term goals that can be easily measured and more quickly achieved. For example, to achieve the long-term goal of transitioning from strained to textured foods, the first step might be to have the patient accept two small bites of a strained food topped with a small amount of dry, finely crushed graham cracker at the beginning of two meals each day. Or, if the goal is to help the patient acquire "beginning" chewing skills (munching movements), the first short-term goal might be to have the patient begin munching activity with a graham cracker placed between the molars (with head and jaw control) two times daily for two bites at lunch time and snack periods. A target period for the achievement of each goal is determined in the evaluation.

Home Program

With the patient and caregiver, I determine the skills that should be practiced at home (e.g., positioning, sensory desensitizing, adapting to new equipment and changes in oral feeding techniques) in order to achieve the patient's goals. Then we discuss and write down the practical details of how, when, where, and how often treatment will be done.

It is very important to emphasize that newly prescribed exercises *should not be done throughout the meal* as the patient may perceive significant differences that are disruptive to the therapeutic process. Snack periods may be used as an appropriate time for practicing techniques as they relieve additional pressure at meal times.

New steps or goals need to be integrated slowly into a treatment program. Patients and caregivers may try too hard to do everything right, which only results in disappointment and failure. The primary goal should be for eating to be safe (no coughing, choking, or aspiration) and provide adequate nutrition. Difficult procedures do not enhance oral intake at first and must be introduced slowly.

It is also important not to introduce too many new techniques at the same time. Caregivers and some patients are wonderfully ambitious and may want to try too many techniques at once. They are often overwhelmed, unsuccessful, and guilt ridden for not accomplishing their goals.

In homes, schools, care facilities, workshops, day programs, and institutions, I always suggest placing the therapeutic home program on a refrigerator with a magnet or taping it to a table or cabinet as a daily reminder. Details are easy to forget if the paper is inside a drawer.

Therapy sessions generally last up to 1 hour. However, in schools or other educational facilities where there are 15 or more students in a room, the sessions must often be abbreviated because of constraints on the amount of time a staff caregiver is able to devote to working with one patient at a time.

Review

I answer all questions and constantly review the hands-on techniques used in therapy so that the caregiver and patient are comfortable with and fully understand each of them. Reviewing the ongoing therapeutic home program at each session provides continuance, comfort, and support and allows the caregiver and patient to discuss changing needs and expectations.

This constant review and assessment can be misinterpreted by caregivers, however. Once, a parent told me that she felt as if I were testing or assessing *her* at each visit. When I heard a similar complaint from a school aide, I realized that I needed to explain the Yossem method more completely to everyone with whom I worked. I emphasize correct performance of the home program so much because success is predicated on a strict adherence to the prescribed techniques that were formulated and written by the patient, caregiver, and myself at each visit.

An important part of reviewing the home program is helping the patient or caregiver recognize the slightest or most subtle sign of progress. Observations such as, "Alicia looked directly at me today," "John opened his mouth one time for me today without any prodding," or "Christie's lips showed a tiny bit of closure on the spoon," are tiny steps of progress that are gratifying to those involved in treatment. I evaluate the results of each therapeutic exercise at every visit and explain that if no progress is seen within a given time we will switch to another therapeutic technique while hopefully maintaining the same treatment goal. It is important that the patient and caregiver feel that there is a beginning and an end to each treatment exercise and that we will never cease looking for (and hopefully finding) new approaches. Any positive change represents success. Regardless of how hopeless the patient or caregiver may feel, I point out the successes (no matter how small) and help them see that there is a "light at the end of the tunnel." To reach that light, it may be necessary to modify our goals or techniques. For this reason, it is very important for me to have organized alternative plans and options.

Problems

Whether I am working with a patient in my private practice or consulting in a facility or school, it is important for me to know why home programs do or do not work as well as anticipated. If the home program does not seem to be working, I first ask if the prescribed exercises were completed. If they were not, I ask the caregiver some or all of the following questions:

Were the exercises asking too much of you (or the patient)?

Were they too difficult or confusing?

Can you demonstrate for me in what part of the exercise the problem occurred?

Did you do the exercises once daily instead of twice (or three times) daily as prescribed?

Did you do the exercises more than the prescribed number of times?

Even though the program may seem to go well initially, new problems may arise during the course of therapy. These problems can be discouraging and defeating when therapy has been going on for many weeks or months. The following questions are appropriate if the patient or caregiver had a particularly difficult week of therapy:

Did you have a bad week (or was the progress the week before so significant that this week's progress was disappointing)?

Did fatigue contribute to your problems?

Were you too busy or ill, or did you just get tired and fed up with the whole routine?

Techniques

Selecting the most productive therapeutic exercise and combining it appropriately with other techniques is the difficult, exciting, and creative part of treatment. For information on the use of specific techniques, see **Part IV**. To select an appropriate technique, I consider the developmental skill required in order for the patient to perform each step in the treatment process as well as the needs of the caregiver. For example, there are several techniques used to develop proper lip closure:

1. An oral conditioning exercise (e.g., lip shaking).
2. Pressure on the tongue with a spoon and simultaneous head flexion.
3. Pressure on the tongue with a spoon without assistive head flexion.

The choice of technique will depend on the developmental skills of the patient. If my patient partially closes his or her lips on a spoon and demonstrates slight head flexion, I would select technique number three. If my patient does not flex his or her head in order to close his or her lips on the spoon, I would select technique number two. I would select technique number one if my patient demonstrates "beginning" movements of lip closure.

When working with children, it is also important to consider how the treatment techniques can be made fun.

Therapists must remember to be flexible. Therapists must bend and sway to accommodate the needs of patients and caregivers while still maintaining treatment continuity. Patients and caregivers become stressed, fatigued, and discouraged after continuous months of therapy. It is up to the therapist to stimulate, motivate, and encourage.

Above all, therapists must remember that there is no cookbook answer.

Signs of Oral Dysfunction

The following is a comprehensive list of signs of oral dysfunction. These signs may appear at any age and be related to many different diagnoses.

- Drooling
- Open-mouth swallowing (i.e., lips and jaws remain open)
- Periods of coughing and choking
- Hypersensitive or hyposensitive gag
- Hyperextension (head thrown back) in swallowing
- "Turkey" swallowing (head flexed downward)
- Tongue thrusts food out of the mouth
- Difficulty with spoon use (raking food off using teeth instead of lips)
- Difficulty eating (or rejection of) textured, chewy foods
- Chewing only in the front or center of the mouth with no lateral movements of tongue or rotary jaw movements
- Sucking movements (see Glossary for definition)
- Messy eating with excessive food and liquid deposited on a bib or apron
- Excessive eating time (often as long as 1 hour per meal)
- Behavioral rigidity (e.g., demanding the same food, plate, or textures daily)
- Meals are unhappy and difficult times for patient, caregiver, or both
- Lack of "cooing" (by 2 months)
- Expressionless face with no fine facial movements
- Drooping eye or corner of the mouth
- No speech or limited speech (in addition to other symptoms)
- Positioning problems (e.g., poor head and trunk control, poor balance, abnormal reflexes)

The following signs may indicate oral dysfunction if they are seen beyond the age at which they would be developmentally normal:

- Eating only pureed, "baby," blended, chopped, or mashed foods
- Drinking from a bottle
- Dribbling when drinking from a cup
- Drinking from a cup with adapted equipment with head hyperextended

Oral-Motor Pre-Speech Feeding Evaluation

The oral-motor pre-speech feeding evaluation consists of physical and behavioral observations made by the therapist or reported by the caregiver or patient. I use the following form when conducting these evaluations. Explanations of normal and abnormal findings follow the form.

Date _____ Patient's Name _____

Age _____ Birth Date _____

Medical Diagnosis _____

_____

Medical History _____

_____

Medications _____

Allergies _____

Behavior (cooperative, resistive, level of awareness) _____

_____

	Legend*	Description
Facial musculature		
Drooling		
Reflex actions		
Rooting reflex		
Suck-swallow reflex		
Bite reflex		
Gag reflex		

*LEGEND: N = normal; ABN = abnormal; BEG = beginning signs; WFL = within functional limits; ABS = absent

	Legend*	Description
Asymmetric tonic neck reflex (ATNR)		
Moro reflex		
Body extension		
Tongue		
Eating		
Not eating		
Jaws		
Eating		
Not eating		
Lips		
Eating		
Not eating		
Response to sensory stimulation		
Outside gums		
On face		
On body		
Within the mouth		
Breathing		
Oral		
Nasal		
Mixed		
Motor speech/voice		
Volume		
Presence of dysarthria		
Language development		
Nonverbal communication		

	Legend*	Description
Dental development		
Bite		
Teeth		
Gums		
Palate		
Posture and feeding position		
Body tone		
Head and trunk control		
Sitting accommodation for feeding		
Feeding behaviors		
Head position		
Body and trunk control		
Swallowing		
Sensory defensiveness		
Biting		
Chewing		
Tongue movements		
Lip movements		
Food consistencies eaten		
Pureed		
Blended		
Mashed with spoon		
Mashed with fork		
Chopped		
Table food (cut up into small pieces)		
Table food (regular-size pieces)		

	Legend*	Description
Feeding patterns		
Number of feeders		
Primary feeder		
Amount of food and liquid intake (24-hour period)		
Preferred foods and liquids		
Preferred textures and temperatures		
Frequency of meals and snacks		
Eagerness to eat		
Length of time to complete a meal or snack		
Atmosphere at meal time		
Independent feeding (if any, with which part of meal?)		
Equipment used		
Spoon_____ Fork_____		
Knife____ Cut-out cup____		
Glass_____ Straw_____		
Cup_____ Bottle_____		
Inner-lip dish_____		
Scoop bowl_____		
Plate guard_____		
Wrist weights_____		
Dycem_____ Apron/bib_____		
Other equipment_____ _____		
Adapted equipment_____		
Need for videofluoroscopic modified barium-swallow evaluation		

Facial musculature
- Normal—face is relaxed with fine movements.
- Abnormal—face demonstrates low or exaggerated muscle tone, abnormal lack of expression, asymmetry, and unrefined movements.

Drooling
- Normal—during teething or when attempting a new activity.
- Abnormal—salivary flow not due to teething; an excessively wet shirt, apron, or bib.

Reflex actions
- Rooting reflex—the head turns toward the food if touched on the cheeks or corners of the mouth. This diminishes at approximately 4 months of age.
- Suck-swallow reflex—anterior and posterior movements of the tongue diminishing at 2–5 months and replaced by the normal suck.

Bite reflex
- Normal—phasic bite begins at approximately 6 months when chewing begins.
- Abnormal—uncontrolled tonic bite; strong biting down on a substance.

Gag reflex
- Normal—protective gag and cough reflex present throughout life.
- Abnormal—placing a finger or spoon further back than ⅔ on the tongue.
- ATNR—a reflex in which the arm extends in the direction in which the head turns. This diminishes at approximately 4–6 months of age.
- Moro—body reacts in extension with abduction of arms and opening of hands to a sudden noise or touch (frequently called a startle reflex). This diminishes at approximately 4–6 months of age.
- Body extension—abnormal thrusting forward and outward movements of the body accompanied by a backward movement of the head.

Tongue
At rest
- Normal—tongue rests quietly within the mouth.
- Abnormal—tongue thrusting, retraction, or deviation.

In motion
- Normal—tongue elevation begins at approximately 6 months. During the chewing process, the tongue laterally transfers food from the sides to the center of the mouth at approximately 7–9 months and across the midline at approximately 12 months. Tongue movements form a groove for liquids and a bolus for foods.
- Abnormal—tongue thrusting or inadequate movements, such as retraction or deviation.

Jaws
At rest (not eating)
- Normal—jaw appears lightly closed.
- Abnormal—jaw may present numerous and varied movements.

In motion (eating)
- Normal—jaw movements begin to stabilize; munching begins at 6 months with lateral movements beginning at approximately 7 months. Vertical, diagonal,

and rotary movements indicate mature chewing ability, which usually develops by 24 months.
- Abnormal—jaw movements vary or may be diminished or absent.

Lips
At rest (not eating)
- Normal—lips are lightly closed and symmetric.
- Abnormal—lips may be open and/or asymmetric.

In motion
- Normal—fine bilabial lip movements can seal the mouth closed at approximately 10–12 months.
- Abnormal—lips may be tense, retracted, or floppy and may not close to form a seal on a cup or spoon.

Sensory defensiveness
- Outside gums—abnormal and excessive reaction or rejection to a firm touch on the gums.
- On face—abnormal rejection of touch on the face, especially around the mouth (the most sensitive part of the body).
- On body—abnormal rejection of touch on varying parts of the body.
- Oral defensiveness—abnormal rejection of textured foods, liquids, or foreign substances.

Breathing
- Oral—abnormal open-mouth breathing (an uncoordinated breathing and swallowing pattern).
- Nasal—normal coordination of breathing and swallowing pattern.
- Mixed—abnormal combination of open- and closed-mouth swallows.

Motor speech/voice
- Loud or soft—hoarse, gravelly sounds may indicate dysfunction at the level of the vocal cords.
- Dysarthria—slurred or imprecise speech can be a result of weakness of the oral musculature and also may relate to poor chewing skills.
- Language—babbling and vocalizing should begin at approximately 2–3 months, one- to two-word utterances at approximately 12 months, and phrases at approximately 2 years.
- Nonverbal communication system—type, how used, how often?
- Body language.
- Cognition—ability to follow directions and answer questions.

Dental development
- Bite (abnormal)—malocclusions (frequently seen in cerebral palsy patients), overbite, underbite.
- Teeth (abnormal)—pointed teeth (as seen in some cerebral palsy patients), unclean appearance (not uncommon in patients with severe oral defensiveness).
- Gums (abnormal)—pale, red, puffy gums (may be due to medication, tactile rejection problems, etc.).
- Palate (abnormal)—high, arched hard palate (frequently seen in cerebral palsy patients); soft palate that does not elevate (can lead to nasal reflux).

I. Background

Posture and feeding position
- Body tone—may be hypertonic, hypotonic, or a combination of both.
- Head and trunk control.
- Type of sitting accommodation used—wheelchair, cut-out table with chair, bed, regular chair, school chair or bench, lap, infant furniture, high chair, etc.

Feeding behaviors (abnormal)
- Head position—head is thrown backward or flexed downward for the swallow.
- Body position—body is incorrectly positioned causing or maintaining excess flexion or extension.
- Swallow—mouth is held open for the swallow and is uncoordinated for the normal breathing and swallowing pattern.
- Sensory defensiveness—rejection of utensils, food, and liquid.
- Biting—unable to bite down on a piece of food or the presence of the tonic bite.
- Chewing—absence of vertical, lateral, or rotary movements.
- Tongue movements—tongue thrust, protrusion, retraction, or inability to control.
- Lip movements—no lip closure on a cup or spoon.
- Spitting.
- Regurgitation.
- Coughing—may occur before, during, or after the swallow.
- Excessive spillage.

Observation for silent aspiration and the need for a videofluoroscopic examination
- Signs to look for—absence of coughing, choking or gagging while swallowing; wet, gurgly sounds; frequent cases of pneumonia or upper respiratory problems.

Feeding Questionnaire for Parents of a Child

1. What particular problem(s) do you feel you have feeding your child? (Parents need to freely express their frustrations, fears, and needs.)
2. What kind of chairs or positions do you use for feeding at home? Do you alternate the use of these?
3. How many bottles (4 or 8 oz) does your child drink per day? (Rather than, "Does your child drink from a bottle?")
4. What time of the day are the bottles given?
5. Does your child use a pacifier?
6. Does your child ever drink from a cup? How much? How often?
7. How long does it take you to feed your child?
8. Who else feeds your child? How often?
9. What liquids does your child drink? (milk, water, juice, soft drinks, etc.)
10. Does your child drool? A lot or a little?
11. Does your child eat only baby or blended table foods?
12. Does your child eat only spoon- or fork-mashed foods or cut-up table foods? (Rather than, "Is your child eating table foods?")
13. Approximately how long has it been since you switched from pureed or baby food to mashed or cut-up fine table foods (if applicable)?
14. Do you give your child snacks? If so, what, when, and how much?
15. Does your child spit out or reject any foods or liquids?
16. What are your child's preferred foods?
17. Does your child cough or choke? If so, when?
18. Does your child attempt finger feeding himself or herself?
19. Does your child attempt to hold the spoon? Do you encourage this?
20. Does your child sit at the table with the rest of the family?
21. What are meal times like? (e.g., hurried, frustrating, difficult, calm, pleasant)
22. Does your child like to eat?
23. Please list everything your child eats and drinks (including specific amounts) for a 3-day period.

Feeding Questionnaire for the Caregiver of an Adult

1. What particular problem(s) do you feel you have feeding your patient (i.e., frustrations, difficulties, needs)?
2. What kind of chair does the patient use when being fed (e.g., regular, wheel-chair, bed)?
3. What kind of chair does the patient use when eating independently?
4. Does the patient use regular or adapted utensils?
5. Does the patient drink from a regular or adapted cup (or glass)? With a straw?
6. Does the patient eat pureed, blended, chopped, or cut-up table food?
7. Does the patient eat snacks? If so, what, when, and how much?
8. What foods and liquids does the patient prefer?
9. How much liquid does the patient drink in a 24-hour period?
10. How many people (in the course of a day) assist the patient with eating?
11. How long does it take to complete a meal?
12. Does the patient like to eat and drink?
13. Does the patient cough, gag, or appear to choke? If so, when?
14. Does the patient eat alone or with family or friends?
15. List everything the patient eats and drinks (including specific amounts) for a 3-day period.

Sensory Defensiveness

In normal development, the sensory system is protective and discriminating. Abnormal development of the sensory system means that the brain is not sending the correct messages to the body letting it know how to integrate the various sensations it receives. This may lead to hypersensitivity (sensory defensiveness) or hyposensitivity to stimuli. These senses often develop before birth. Hyposensitivity and hypersensitivity may be at least partially responsible for some feeding disorders and need to be addressed early in the course of therapy. Patients of all ages may be so hypersensitive to touch that it becomes a major barrier to use of many therapy techniques and personal interactions. It is vital that patients accept touch (at least on the torso, shoulders, and head) before feeding therapy can begin. For example, pressure on the tongue with the bowl of the spoon is a technique used to stimulate lip closure. A patient with hypersensitivity, however, would not allow this intrusion. A patient with hyposensitivity might place the spoon further back into the mouth than is safe.

Treatment of hypersensitivity emphasizes sensory desensitizing of the entire body, beginning with the extremities and moving toward the face and the mouth (the most sensitive part of the body). I have found brisk towel rubbing to be the most successful treatment for hypersensitivity to touch. The firm, deep pressure appears to decrease uncomfortable and distressful feelings while a light touch causes a negative response. For more information on specific treatment techniques, see **Part IV**.

Because sensory defensiveness may be a serious problem, it is important to understand its complexities and its relationship to feeding problems. A. Jean Ayres has published numerous articles and books on this topic. The following abbreviated case studies highlight the importance of decreasing sensory defensiveness.

CASE STUDY 1

> The regional center for the handicapped schools of Los Angeles asked me to visit the home of Jennifer, who was 1 year old at the time. I was told only that she was developmentally delayed and that her main problem was a refusal to eat anything other than a little strained food. She had no known physical problems and received no medication. Her two siblings ate normally and her parents were naturally very concerned.
>
> During my initial evaluation, I observed Jennifer sitting on an uncarpeted section of the floor in the living room as

she closely watched my every move. Her mother had placed numerous toys around her. When I sat down to play with Jennifer, she completely rejected the toys as well as my touch. When her mother joined us, Jennifer also rejected her efforts. Her mother told me that Jennifer preferred plastic or wooden toys (nothing fuzzy or cuddly) and disliked being handled or caressed, even by her parents and siblings. She would not even sit on the carpet unless she was wearing long pants and long sleeves. Attempts to feed Jennifer textured food were disastrous. She ate strained baby food, but only in small amounts because she appeared to hate having a spoon in her mouth. Obviously, part of Jennifer's problem was sensory defensiveness.

After I explained sensory desensitization techniques to Jennifer's mother and father, we wrote up a home program of therapeutic exercises together. Tactile rubbing (see Part IV) was begun immediately. Approximately 3 weeks later, we began using gentle pressure with a spoon on the tongue. In 2 months, Jennifer was eating well, playing with all types of toys, and enjoying limited cuddling.

CASE STUDY 2

I was invited to give a lecture on the Yossem method of feeding therapy to a group of parents who all had very young children who regurgitated or rejected food and were irritable and difficult to manage. My short presentation followed a lecture by a highly recognized physician who explained that in his practice he found many children who were fussy eaters and that since these children had all been evaluated and no physical problems could be seen, his solution was to expose them more frequently to normal children at snack and mealtimes.

After much thought and observation of the parents' discomfort with these statements, I decided to begin my talk with the following questions: (1) Do your children prefer long sleeves and long pants? (2) Do they enjoy playing with fuzzy, cuddly toys? I shall never forget the look on those parents' faces—what did these questions have to do with feeding and regurgitation? However, just as I expected, they all responded affirmatively to the first question and negatively to the second. I explained that some people dislike or reject exposure to any type of touch, such as the touch of a hand, certain types of clothing, fuzzy toys, grass, or carpeting. These people will also frequently reject a spoon in the mouth and textured foods. This causes feeding problems and may create havoc for the patient and the family.

I am happy to report that the children whose parents followed various therapeutic suggestions ceased regurgitation after their second visit to my office. After a few sessions of rubbing techniques and individualized feeding therapy techniques, food acceptance began. All patients progressed at a slow but very satisfactory rate. I felt comforted and encouraged by these results, as eating time became more pleasurable for the children and their families.

Positioning

DEVELOPMENT OF MOVEMENT

The development of movement follows a fairly characteristic pattern in normal people. Head balance is acquired between birth and 2 months and rolling at 2–4 months. Most infants sit with assistance at 5–7 months and without assistance at approximately 6–9 months as they are able to rotate and move from supine to prone to sitting positions. Sitting is followed by crawling, kneeling, standing, and walking. These actions are possible because children learn how to maintain proper body alignment and to stabilize specific movements (independent of other movements). For example, head motions can be initiated without turning the rest of the body. The mouth can be opened and closed in a controlled pattern. Children soon learn the process of closing the lips, stabilizing the cup, and drinking without throwing the rest of the body out of alignment.

DEVELOPMENT OF MOVEMENT IN INDIVIDUALS WITH DISABILITIES

The acquisition of good or adequate body positioning is the primary focus in helping physically handicapped persons acquire normal movement skills. Normal standing position, for example, requires that the body is positioned so that the head and arms are midline; the body, feet, and head stabilized to avoid excess flexion or extension (backward movement); and the shoulders protracted with a slightly flexed neck.

Elimination of abnormal reflexes (e.g., the Moro and extension reflex) helps to improve balance and attention span and is, therefore, also important in working with persons with disabilities. It is difficult for a person to pay attention to skill acquisition when he or she feels insecure about body positioning. When a person feels that his or her body is no longer a burden that is difficult to control, the rate of motor development will increase. Gross and fine motor skills can be better learned if the person feels that arms and hands can be used independently from the sides of the body without losing his or her center of gravity.

MOVEMENT AND POSITIONING IN FEEDING THERAPY

Abnormal muscle tone and movement generally involves the entire body and affects feeding and swallowing. Working to attain proper positioning despite abnormal muscle tone and control is, therefore, a vital part of feeding therapy. Incorrect positioning may be responsible for feeding problems and may make swallowing unsafe. I have treated hundreds of patients with upper motor neuron problems (e.g., cerebral palsy) that require intensive positioning adaptations in all kinds of chairs, recliners, and beds. Therapeutic positioning may help to do the following:

- Normalize muscle tone
- Decrease the influence of pathologic reflexes
- Decrease the tendency toward contractures (tightening of the muscles)
- Increase stability
- Maximize functional activity
- Facilitate relaxation

The amount and type of body support required for proper positioning varies according to the individual patient. Hypertonic patients, for example, generally demonstrate patterns of flexion or extension while hypotonic patients generally demonstrate slower, more floppy movements. A severely involved patient with hypotonia may require a slightly reclined chair and a small foam block under the hips. A hypertonic patient may require a larger and more dense foam block under the hips. The size of the foam block placed at the nape of the neck varies according to the individual's need. While movement activities are encouraged to improve general muscle tone whenever possible at other times of the day, stabilization is vital during feeding. However, stabilization does not mean that the patient is rigid in the chair. Space for some movement should be available. The primary aim of stabilization is to decrease the effort required by the patient during the eating and swallowing process. Because all body parts are interconnected and must work together, poor control of trunk, hip, and pelvic movements affects purposeful body, head, neck, and oral control. Inadequate stabilization also affects breathing and swallowing whether the head is in hyperextension or hyperflexion.

I have found that it is best to prepare infants and children for the feeding position by using the positioning chair for play or relaxation activities. This helps them associate the chair with positive interaction and they are more likely to accept its use during feeding. Other techniques, such as cradling a child whose body is held in extension before placement in a chair, may help to relax the child and ease his or her adjustment to the positioning chair.

I frequently position patients in an almost upright position. Patients with diminished or "floppy" tone, however, may require a slightly reclined position because a fully upright posture may cause their head to fall backward (or forward) and their mouth to fall open. Sitting position is actually determined by the position and stability of the hips, trunk control, and pelvis. This varies with each patient. The hips and knees should be flexed to approximately 60–75 degrees to inhibit extensor tone. A foam wedge (uncovered to prevent slipping and washable) placed under the buttocks can help provide additional hip flexion if needed. The tallest part of the wedge is placed under the knees. Shifting of body weight off of the spine and onto the buttocks is vital. Feet need to be stabilized (Figure 1). Shoulders should be moved into a slightly protracted position (using foam wedges if necessary) to prevent hyperextension of the head and neck and to encourage purposeful arm movements.

Pressure on the back of the head may create hyperextension in some cases (e.g., in patients with spastic cerebral palsy). A foam wedge or towel should be placed at the nape of the neck to counteract this tendency. When shoulders are abnormally retracted, tongue, jaw, and lip movements are also negatively affected. It is especially important to correctly position the head, neck, and chin to provide align-

Figure 1
Positioning with foam
blocks.

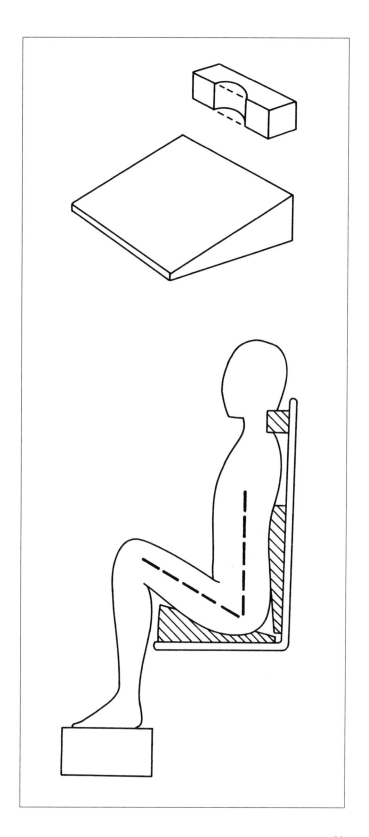

ment for safe swallowing. Head and neck stability depends on body tone, shoulder positioning, and hip and trunk control. Hyperextension may allow food or liquid to enter the trachea, causing coughing, choking, and perhaps aspiration. It is also extremely important to be aware of the possibility of silent aspiration.

The following adaptive sitting positions all offer therapeutic body positioning, excellent eye contact (with the exception of a few types of wheelchairs), stabilization, safety, and comfort for persons of all ages with varying problems.

Infants

- Reclining on the lap (facing the caregiver) supported with a pillow or a wedge
- Sitting on the lap
- Prone on a wedge on a table
- Prone on the lap
- Car seats
- Infant seats

Children

- Feeding chairs
- Corner chairs or bolster chairs
- Travel chairs
- Cut-out tables and chairs
- School chairs
- Tumble-form chairs
- Modular seating arrangements
- Wheelchairs
- Standing tables (prone boards)
- Car seats

Adults

- Wheelchairs
- Prone standers and boards
- Cut-out tables and chairs
- Large, circular tables accommodating four to six adults in wheelchairs
- Bed positioning for persons unable to sit in a chair

It is still frequently necessary to adapt chairs using pillows, head and side supports, foam wedges, towels, abductor wedges (to separate the legs), or adductor wedges (to bring the legs closer together). All adaptations need to provide stability and control of the body and head as well as fine motor control for independent eating (when possible). It may be necessary to change or modify positioning in the chair to accommodate growth or changes in movement and contractures.

Basic Hierarchy of Foods

CHOOSING FOODS

Food consistency and nutrition are important considerations for all patients with feeding disorders. Menus can become bland and boring for patients who are unable to chew. Poor food choices that do not take into account the needs of the individual patient can cause further problems during feeding, including coughing, choking, gagging, and aspiration. If patients become fearful of eating because they have had difficulty with inappropriate foods or feel rushed or tense during eating, they may begin rejecting food altogether. The hierarchy or order of foods that we offer our patients is vital in that it determines the way the patient begins to develop his or her eating and drinking skills.

Foods that are too thin, too thick, too sticky (e.g., peanut butter), or of mixed consistencies (e.g., soup with vegetables) are often inappropriate for persons with feeding disorders. The following factors should be taken into account when deciding on the appropriateness of a certain food:

- What is its nutritional value? (Consultation with a nutritionist may be helpful in planning menus.)
- What is its texture, size, and weight?
- What is its consistency (e.g., smooth, lumpy, or grainy)?
- Is it chopped, mashed, cut up, or pureed?
- What happens to it when it mixes with saliva (e.g., white bread turns into paste)?
- Is it likely to get stuck on the hard palate or between the molars (e.g., peanut butter)?
- Does it provide auditory feedback (crunchy foods) or is it stringy and slippery (e.g., cantaloupe; long, thin green beans)?
- Does it combine two textures (some "junior" foods, soups) making a patient wonder whether to suck, sip, or chew?
- Does it taste bland or flavorful? (Added seasonings are enticing to many patients who appear to have diminished taste buds.)
- Does it have an odor?
- What does it look like? (Presentation does matter.)
- What is its temperature?
- Is the food similar to those eaten at home?

It is also important to consider a food's therapeutic value and whether it requires the patient to work on the development of specific skills such as biting down or rotational chewing. Food choice may be guided in part by whether the patient is working on acceptance of new textures, improvement of tongue movements (vertical or lateral), improvement of lip closure, jaw movements, or liquid intake. The therapist and caregiver should also consider whether the patient is able to purposefully use his or her lips, tongue, and jaw in a meaningful, comfortable, and safe manner when chewing or drinking a specific food or liquid. An incorrect choice of foods only facilitates abnormal movements and, therefore, does not help to correct inadequate oral musculature.

DECREASING SENSITIVITY AND RESISTANCE TO TEXTURED FOODS

One of the most important components of therapy for many patients with feeding disorders is decreasing sensitivity to and resistance or rejection of textured foods. I use the following series of steps to achieve decreased sensitivity with my patients:

1. Begin thickening blended or pureed foods by adding a small amount of finely crushed graham crackers or baby cereal.
2. When the patient comfortably accepts this mixture, add a little more graham in gradual steps until the food is the texture of oatmeal.
3. Add small, then medium, and finally large pieces of graham folded into each individual bite. It is advisable to have graham pieces prepared in advance in separate containers.
4. Sprinkle finely crushed graham on top of the bites with the graham folded in.
5. Add a few large pieces of graham on top of the bites.
6. Introduce soft, textured table foods.

These initial steps may take anywhere from 1 week to 1 month or more depending on the diagnosis of the patient and the consistency of care. To introduce textured foods, I incorporate the following hierarchical sequence of foods:

1. Cooked carrot or potato; tips of cooked broccoli, asparagus, or cauliflower; beets; soup vegetables; avocado; fresh pear; banana; and egg salad with a tiny bit of mayonnaise (all mashed with a fork).
2. The foods above with the addition of soft casseroles, scrambled eggs, *canned* pears, tuna salad with mayonnaise, soft quiches, and jarred gefilte fish (all mashed with a spoon).

TEACHING CHEWING SKILLS

The proper choice of foods for teaching chewing skills is vital. Foods should have a texture that stimulates biting motions but are not slippery, too hard, or bulky. The sequence of foods I frequently use is as follows:

1. Graham cracker (I find most other crackers to be too crispy or hard. Sensitive patients frequently object to sharp edges.)
2. Cooked, soft, solid potato, carrots, or kidney beans
3. Wide, long, puffy cheese puffs (an encouraging auditory feedback)

4. Fresh pear cube and crispy watermelon cube
5. Jicama or wide, lightly cooked green beans
6. Tiny cubes of soft, solid cooked chicken; fish; or cubed sandwich meat

The following foods should *not* be used for teaching and practicing chewing skills because they do not encourage good biting movements or tongue lateralization and may be swallowed whole:

- Canned peaches (too slippery and usually swallowed whole)
- Fruit cocktail (never chewed and generally swallowed as soon as it is placed into the mouth)
- Cantaloupe and banana (too slippery and therefore difficult to bite down on or to chew)
- Stringy green beans (too thin to manipulate and may be swallowed whole)
- Banana (too soft to bite down on)
- Hamburger and apple (dissipate all over the mouth, making it difficult to form a bolus)
- Chips and raw carrots and celery (too hard)
- Sandwich-meat strips and American cheese strips (usually swallowed in one piece)
- Stringy chicken and beef (too difficult to manipulate)

INTRODUCING LIQUIDS

Thickened liquids, such as juice thickened with runny applesauce, plain yogurt that has been stirred well to a thinned consistency, strained baby foods, and cream soups, are often easiest for patients who are just beginning to drink. The amount of thickening agent may be decreased slowly until the patient is ready to attempt liquids such as apricot or nectar juice and finally, water. Small, slow sips reduce coughing and the possibility of choking.

ADDITIONAL PRECAUTIONS

Schools and adult residential facilities for those individuals with disabilities have requested that I provide a list of foods that should never be eaten by patients with feeding, chewing, or swallowing problems. If swallowed whole, these foods may block the trachea and compromise the person's breathing. The following list has been posted in classrooms, dining rooms, or day rooms and has served as a simple but effective reminder of precautions.

- Popcorn
- Nuts
- Hard candies
- Chewy candies
- Jelly beans
- Dates
- Marshmallows

- Raisins (uncooked)
- Dried fruits
- Peanut butter (creates abnormal sucking movements and excess saliva)
- Stringy foods
- Chicken or beef strips (small chunks are fine)
- Menudo
- Lettuce salad (finely diced with mayonnaise is acceptable)
- Sticky, dry foods
- Hot dogs (unless finely diced)
- Raw vegetables such as carrots and celery (unless finely diced)
- Fruits such as apples with skin, large slices of orange, chunks of cantaloupe, whole grapes, unpitted cherries, canned pineapple chunks, canned peaches.
- Plastic utensils (easily broken and swallowed with food)
- Hamburger and apple (tend to break up and scatter within the mouth; hamburger is best mixed with ketchup, salsa, or mayonnaise to make it more cohesive)
- Sandwich meat or American cheese slices (unless cubed)
- Fruit cocktail (may be acceptable if mashed with a fork and served in small portions)
- White bread (when mixed with saliva it sticks to the hard palate in clumps)
- Tortillas (may be too dry, hard, bulky, or sticky)
- A healthy way to offer fresh fruits and vegetables with the pulp is to blend them into whipped gelatin.

In a school or other care institution, it is helpful to post a chart so staff members are familiar with the types of food and adaptations needed for each individual patient.

Name	Food Texture	Adaptive Equipment	Hand Usage
John	Regular (cut-up)	Plate guard; cut-out cup	Left
Mary	Mashed with fork	Cut-out cup; dycem (a table mat that sticks to a table or tray)	Right
Jill	Regular	Fork; knife; glass	Left
Beau	Mashed (breads should be soaked)	Straw; cup holder	Must be assisted
Jamie	Regular	Scoop bowl or plate guard; large spoon; straw in a tall glass; lap tray	Left
Alice	Mashed with fork and moistened	Universal cuff on right wrist; scoop bowl; small glass	Right

II
Case Studies: Private Practice

The Case of the University Professor: A Sudden Swallowing Problem

DESCRIPTION AND PRESENTING PROBLEM

Dorothy, an attractive, intelligent 40-year-old university professor, came to my office hoping that I could help solve feeding problems that she had been experiencing for 9 years. Her main problems were frequent coughing and gagging. She wondered if she would "ever be able to enjoy food like other normal people." Because of her feeding problems, she avoided social situations that involved eating. At her university office, she ate privately so no one could see or hear her. She frequently spit food into her napkin because she could not swallow it without coughing.

I asked Dorothy to tell me when her problems began. "In 1984, I was attending a national conference and just before my presentation I sat down to lunch," she said. "Suddenly, I could not swallow! I tried again and again but to no avail. Up to this point I had been a voracious eater, so this was very unusual." The problem continued and after several weeks Dorothy made appointments at Harvard University. She consulted with two physicians and x-rays were taken. She was told that her problem was not mechanical in nature. Believing the problem might be related to stress, she tried several months of psychotherapy, in which she was told her problem was not psychological. In the late 1980s, she sought help from a neurologist, an acupuncturist, and a hypnotherapist.

FIRST VISIT

The pre-speech, oral-motor feeding evaluation indicated the following dysfunctions:

Dysfunction	Explanation
Excessive head flexion for each swallow of food or liquid	Flexion and "pushing the food downward" helped Dorothy to swallow her food, which could not be swallowed normally be-

Dysfunction	Explanation
	cause of inadequate tongue movements.
A sip of liquid, preferably milk, was used to "push each bite down"	Liquid was used to help the food "slide down" to compensate for inadequate tongue movement.
Abnormal tongue movements are used for chewing	Dorothy was apparently unable to form a bolus with her tongue and could not easily propel the food to the posterior region for the swallow.
Frequent, small coughs	Instead of forming a bolus with the tongue, the food would spread out into Dorothy's mouth and into the trachea causing little coughs. Once the food entered the pharynx, everything proceeded normally.
Excessive chewing of each bite	This time was spent trying to gather the food into a cohesive bolus, manipulate it about, and swallow it.
Mixed swallows	Dorothy alternated between normal coordinated swallows and abnormal uncoordinated swallows.
Spitting out food into a napkin after excessive chewing	When Dorothy found she could not gather all of the food together into a bolus to swallow or the food made her "uncomfortable," she would spit the food into the napkin as gracefully as possible
Food preferences were rice, crispy bacon, toast, and cookies (all soft foods had been eliminated)	Soft foods frightened Dorothy because they "slid down too rapidly." She could not shape her tongue around the soft food because of abnormal and inefficient tongue movements.

To confirm my "bedside" diagnosis that Dorothy was not aspirating food or liquid, a videofluoroscopy (modified barium swallow) was arranged at the local hospital with a radiologist and speech-language pathologist in attendance. The report stated that "the overall swallow function was abnormal and characterized by delayed oral preparation, decreased anterior to posterior propulsion of the bolus through the oral cavity, and normal pharyngeal motility into the esophagus. Premature spillage of liquids into the hypopharynx was present. No aspiration of any consistency was noted. Speech, intelligence, and articulation were within normal limits." A neurologic examination was suggested and completed shortly thereafter. It showed no hypoglossal nerve dysfunction. No problem at the level of the vocal cords was found. No diagnosis or suggested treatment was given.

Goals

Although no specific medical diagnosis was made in Dorothy's case, I did not consider this a deterrent to setting up a treatment program. As there were no health problems that would interfere with the swallowing treatment program, Dorothy and I agreed on the following treatment goals.

Long-Term Goals

- To swallow all food and liquids without any problem
- To chew normally

Short-Term Goals

- To alleviate fear of eating
- To inspire confidence by establishing the comfort zone for therapy
- To retrain the tongue muscles to prepare the food bolus
- To decrease mastication time and excessive tongue and jaw movements
- To accept varying textures of food
- To relearn a normal, coordinated swallow

INTERVENTIONS

All visits were weeks apart due to the patient's erratic work and travel schedule.

SECOND VISIT (1 WEEK LATER)

I began with casual conversation to create a relaxed atmosphere. Next, as I did at each following visit, I observed Dorothy feed herself before I offered food and liquid to her. Dorothy was eager to begin therapy and was comfortable with the following suggestions for the home program.

Home Program	Rationale
Practice two or three saliva swallows (without food) twice daily. I instructed Dorothy to place her tongue on the hard	This exercise simulates a normal coordinated swallow. Dorothy is able to feel safe and in control because no

Home Program	Rationale
palate, close her jaw and lips, and swallow her saliva.	food is used, eliminating the fear of coughing.
Perform swallows with a tiny bit of soft but textured food, using the procedure above. I asked Dorothy to use apple-sauce thickened with crushed graham crackers when she felt she could try this without too much anxiety. I instructed her to not use liquid to push the food down.	This food combination is fairly easy for Dorothy to work with because it is smooth but tex-tured and encourages her to use her tongue to gather the food into a bolus before the swallow.
(Both exercises could be done during dinner at home and between her classes.)	

THIRD VISIT (1 WEEK LATER)

Dorothy began by telling me about her progress. She thought she was moving ahead too slowly (after only *two* visits). I explained that she could expect to see small steps of progress frequently, but not major changes this soon. We laughed to-gether and continued.

Next, I observed Dorothy eating the preferred textured foods she had brought. I observed her discomfort as she ate the soft foods I offered her—thickened apple-sauce, yogurt, and a soft cookie. In between her bites we chatted about everyday things, *not* about food.

Because our casual conversation made Dorothy comfortable, I was able to observe her automatic swallows. When I next told Dorothy that we would not talk while I watched her eating her preferred food, her swallowing responses while she ate be-came exacerbated. Her swallow was accompanied by excess head flexion (when swallowing liquids), tiny coughs, and the need to spit out her food. When Dorothy was unaware of being watched, she swallowed more easily, had less coughing, and slightly less mastication preceding the swallow. When I shared my observations with Dorothy, she was encouraged and excited to know she was already making im-provements. I instructed her to work on the following exercises until our next visit.

Home Program	Rationale
Continue the exercises pre-scribed at the second visit with less thickening of the applesauce.	Dorothy needed to be shown again how to use her tongue correctly for the coordinated swallows.
Incorporate the saliva swallow exercise into traveling time in the car.	Performing exercises alone in the car allows privacy and increased practice time.

Home Program	Rationale
Concentrate on head position while swallowing liquids.	Dorothy needed to learn how little flexion is actually required to swallow liquids.
Concentrate on taking small bites of food and eating more slowly.	I knew that Dorothy would be leaving soon on a business trip. I hoped that these suggestions would alleviate some of her fear of eating and drinking in public and decrease excessive chewing motions.

FOURTH VISIT (1 MONTH LATER)

I had not seen Dorothy for 1 month because she was traveling abroad to conduct research. On her return, she told me that she had eaten more food on the plane than ever before! She also drank milk (her preference) and was careful not to flex her head excessively. Dorothy's attempt to eat new foods in public indicated increasing confidence and understanding of her problem. She remembered to take small bites and to eat slowly to decrease coughing and the need to spit out her food. However, she still had "crisis times" in which she coughed, became frightened, and was unable to continue eating. During this visit, I observed improved mastication (and, therefore, less required chewing time), few little coughs, less head flexion, and more coordinated swallows. The reason for the crises was undetermined; it is possible that anxiety could have been a precipitating factor during the time abroad. The following home program exercises were assigned.

Home Program	Rationale
Continue saliva swallows two to three times daily, especially when experiencing difficulty eating.	Saliva swallows are calming (see second visit). After rebuilding confidence, Dorothy will feel better eating the preferred food.
Take smaller bites of food than usual.	It is easier to chew, form a bolus, and swallow with smaller amounts of food. This should also decrease coughing.
Avoid using liquid to assist with the swallows. The cup of milk should be kept at arm's length and only used for emergencies.	Dorothy needs to learn to chew and swallow without liquids to "push food down." Knowing that liquid is within reach helps her feel more comfortable.
Introduce a smooth food. Dorothy chose yogurt with	At this point in therapy, eating a smooth food would cause a

Home Program	Rationale
crumbled saltines as a thickening agent. She was to take five bites from the spoon (¼ teaspoon) twice daily. Each day Dorothy was encouraged to decrease the amount of thickening until she was able to accept a smooth consistency.	return to the dysfunctional symptoms. Therefore, it was best to add a thickening substance. I cautioned Dorothy not to move too rapidly. Though she was eager to progress, moving too quickly could cause regression.

FIFTH VISIT (2 WEEKS LATER)

Dorothy informed me that she continued to have crises. She also "forgets" her instructions and occasionally uses water or milk to assist in eating textured foods. She was delighted that she was eating more, becoming more adventurous in her choice of foods, and gaining weight. Best of all, she felt secure enough to begin eating once again in social situations and at work. She stopped eating only when she thought that people might be looking at her.

Dorothy was unaware that I was closely observing her eating and swallowing skills while we talked. I noted fewer excessive chewing and tongue movements with each bite and practically no abnormal head flexion or coughs. When I informed her that I would be observing her eating skills, she reverted to the exaggerated movements. We discussed the following steps to be implemented in the home program.

Home Program	Rationale
Continue the saliva swallow exercise with additional practice time daily.	Encouraged by her success, Dorothy was eating rapidly and practicing her yogurt exercise too often. Continuing the saliva exercise reminds her to slow down and follow the steps of the coordinated swallow.
Place the cup of liquid at the opposite end of the table (Dorothy's suggestion).	The presence of the liquid helps alleviate Dorothy's fears. It cannot, however, be used as a crutch when the cup is placed out of her reach.
Practice tucking in the chin with simultaneous head flexion for each swallow (Figure 2).	This chin tuck position is a good way for Dorothy to remember to use only slight head flexion for swallowing liquids.
Continue the exercise using thickened smooth yogurt (re-	The thickened yogurt needs to be thinner so that progress to

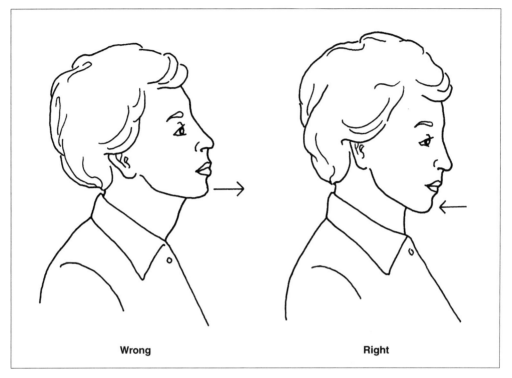

Wrong	Right

Figure 2
Examples of correct and incorrect chin-tuck positions.

Home Program	Rationale
duced now to the consistency of runny oatmeal) three to five times per day with ¼ teaspoon portions.	ward eating smooth food continues. We prepared the food together at this visit to ensure that Dorothy knew the proper texture.

SIXTH VISIT (2 WEEKS LATER)

Because she was busy preparing for another trip abroad for her research, Dorothy had reduced the number of times she practiced her exercises. She was now only doing them during her crises. We thoroughly discussed when, how, and what Dorothy thought she could accomplish while she was away, and the following home program was outlined.

Home Program	Rationale
Continue the saliva swallows as often as possible.	This will promote further skill integration and swallowing comfort.

Home Program	Rationale
Continue thinning the cracker-thickened yogurt or applesauce (whichever is available at the time) with water or milk.	This will help Dorothy continue to accept smoother foods.
Take smaller bites of textured foods.	This will reduce excessive chewing movements, remind Dorothy to place her tongue correctly, and slow the pace of eating.

SEVENTH VISIT (2 MONTHS LATER)

Dorothy returned from her trip inspired by her success. She had been able to eat with her colleagues and to thoroughly enjoy herself. She claimed she was eating "everything in sight." She had, however, become overconfident and decreased the number of times she performed her exercises. I observed both positive and negative developments. Dorothy was excessively flexing her head again with each swallow of liquid, using liquids more frequently to push food down, and eating too rapidly. Mastication time was shortened, however, and the coughing had ceased. She ate a hamburger during our session to demonstrate her success. She did not cough or spit out food at all. We agreed to work on decreasing the excessive head flexion and the use of liquid to assist in swallowing.

Home Program	Rationale
Continue the saliva exercise while maintaining an almost upright head position (slight flexion with the chin tuck).	Integration and reinforcement
Continue thickening yogurt with only a small amount of crushed cracker.	Continue progress toward accepting smooth foods.
Practice the coordinated swallow with a drop of plain, smooth yogurt.	Integration

EIGHTH VISIT (1 WEEK LATER)

Therapy exercises were practiced half-heartedly this past week. Dorothy and I talked about the need for consistency, especially when so much progress is being made.

Home Program	Rationale
Eat ¼ of a meal (three times daily when possible) maintain-	Promote awareness so consistency can be achieved.

Figure 3
Application of cup pressure on the bottom lip.

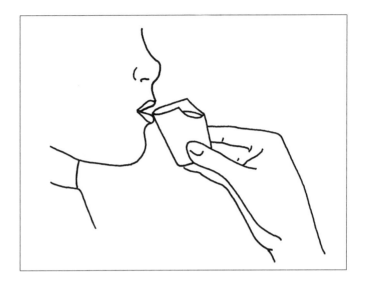

Home Program	Rationale
ing awareness of head and tongue positioning and eating small bites of food.	
Place a cup containing very runny, plain yogurt on the bottom lip. Hold it there while drinking a tiny sip followed quickly by two more sips. This should be repeated twice two to three times daily (Figure 3).	This quick swallow exercise hastens abnormally slow swallows. The added pressure of the cup on the lower lip makes it easier to swallow the yogurt.
Continue to place the cup of emergency milk out of reach. A drink may be taken halfway through the meal	This will continue to provide comfort (but not a crutch) for Dorothy.

NINTH VISIT (1 MONTH LATER)

Dorothy requested this delayed visit. She wanted to concentrate on doing her therapy exercises at home for an extended period. She is very determined to "work hard and finish up." She is doing quite well today and coordinated swallows with smooth yogurt appear to be improving.

Home Program	Rationale
Continue the quick swallow exercise and place the cup of emergency liquid out of reach.	Integration and awareness

The Case of the University Professor: A Sudden Swallowing Problem

TENTH VISIT (1 WEEK LATER)

Cup drinking speed appears normal and coordinated. Food consumption is excellent with no excessive chewing or tongue movements before the swallows. However, I still see some excess head flexion when Dorothy swallows liquid, especially when she is fatigued. (I frequently see Dorothy after she finishes teaching her classes.)

Home Program	Rationale
Continue the quick swallow exercise.	This will maintain quick (and now normal) swallows and the coordinated swallow.
Continue to be aware of chewing and tongue movements.	Maintenance of awareness
Keep the cup of liquid out of reach during meals.	Dorothy still thinks she needs liquid to swallow her food.

ELEVENTH VISIT (2 WEEKS LATER)

Dorothy tells me that she has returned to eating smooth chocolate pudding, thin oatmeal, chocolate mousse, and other smooth foods. She is extremely happy but is worried that she will have to watch her diet! I did not observe any excess head flexion while she was eating and drinking. She is not having any crisis times. Everything seems to be going well.

Home Program	Rationale
Continue the exercises from the tenth visit.	Maintenance

TWELFTH VISIT (3 WEEKS LATER)

Dorothy continues to enjoy all foods, even soft textures, but admits that she has neglected the prescribed exercises. Once again, I observe excess head flexion while she is drinking. It is not uncommon for a patient who is comfortable with successes and has no discomfort to decrease practice time and experience relapses.

Home Program	Rationale
Position elbows on the table, place left index finger under the lower lip and middle finger under chin. The right hand will hold the cup lightly on the lower lip while Dorothy takes small sips of milk and swallows	Another new exercise. This independent head and jaw stabilization eliminates excessive head flexion. Remembering to use the chin tuck did not provide significant improvement. Hopefully, Dorothy will be

Figure 4
Use of the controlled hand position for independent head and jaw stabilization.

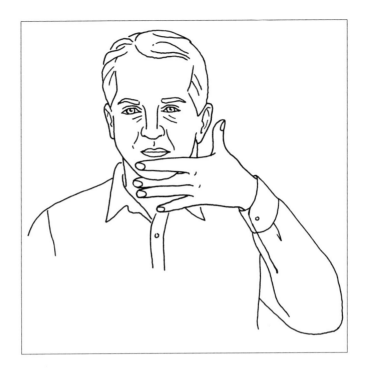

Home Program	Rationale
with closed lips. This exercise should be performed at breakfast and in the early evening (Figure 4).	able to stop using this assistive help within 1–2 weeks. I chose these times for use of the technique to account for morning overenthusiam and to compensate for evening fatigue.
Stop practicing the quick swallow exercise.	The speed of swallowing now appears to be normal (a great goal met).

THIRTEENTH VISIT (1 WEEK LATER)

Dorothy continues to demonstrate excellent progress.

Home Program	Rationale
Practice independent head and jaw stabilization.	Continuation and maintenance
Practice saliva swallows three times daily in the car and at home in the evening.	Because this exercise can be done easily at different times, it encourages ongoing coordinated swallows.

FOURTEENTH VISIT (1 WEEK LATER)

Practice times have been going well. Dorothy is very pleased with the results.

Home Program	Rationale
Begin drinking using cognitive awareness instead of the head and jaw stabilization techniques.	Continued progression
Continue saliva swallows.	Maintenance

FIFTEENTH VISIT (1 WEEK LATER)

Dorothy tells me she only rarely reaches for the cup of liquid during meals. Usually, her need for liquid appears to be stress related. Head positioning is much improved with infrequent moments of excessive flexion.

CONCLUSION

Practice is all that Dorothy requires to complete her therapy. I, therefore, suggest that we keep in touch through phone calls. Dorothy has her ups and downs but is comfortable because she knows what she has to do to take care of herself.

Length of intervention: 8 months, 15 visits.

The Case of the Musician: Jaw Surgery Following a Motor Vehicle Accident

DESCRIPTION AND PRESENTING PROBLEM

Thomas requested my help in treating his severe feeding and swallowing problems in January 1982. These problems as well as other neuromuscular difficulties forced him to stay at home and be fed by a nasogastric tube. He required constant nursing care. Thomas was a charming, intelligent, and creative 70 year old. He had composed songs and conducted orchestras for well-known stars and Broadway shows. Being "tied down" to his home and unable to work only increased his tension and exacerbated his swallowing problems.

Thomas had undergone jaw surgery for a bilateral mandibular fracture following a severe motor vehicle accident the previous year. Soon after surgery he developed feeding and swallowing problems that appeared to be unrelated to the trauma from the accident. Even though his physicians made no definitive diagnosis of his feeding problems, they noted that Thomas did have a "primary disease affecting his tongue." Thomas told me that he had consulted with 18 physicians but that no further diagnosis was made and no treatment was offered. His physician discussed the case with a speech-language pathologist who recommended me. He finally agreed to let Thomas work with me. Treatment began after approval was received from Thomas's oral surgeons.

FIRST VISIT

The pre-speech, oral-motor feeding evaluation indicated the following dysfunctions.

Dysfunction	Explanation
Inadequate lip and jaw closure	Thomas has decreased muscle tone with limited oral-motor control.

Dysfunction	Explanation
Excessive, constant drooling	Because his mouth is open all of the time, loss of saliva and drooling occur. Inadequate motor control of tongue, jaw, and lip movements combined with the open mouth allowed loss of saliva and drooling.
Diminished sensation in tongue and lips	Diminished tactile sensation due to Thomas's neurologic problems.
Delayed gag	Due to his neurologic problems, I was able to "walk" further back on the tongue with my finger than the normal ⅔ distance.
Abnormal (diminished) tongue movements	Thomas has problems moving his tongue from side to center or side to side due to decreased muscle control.
No jaw rotation for chewing	Thomas only moves his tongue and jaw in limited up-and-down vertical movements due to decreased muscle control.
Inability to swallow food and liquid	Total absence of oral-motor control due to neurologic problems.
Tactile defensiveness within the oral area	Thomas does not wish to be touched by utensils or textured food within his mouth due to sensory defensiveness arising from his neurologic problems.
No speech	No medical diagnosis has been determined at this time. Thomas writes with pen and paper to communicate.

The nasogastric tube delivered feedings to Thomas five times a day. Because he was unable to control his saliva, suction was used frequently by the nurses. A bib apron was worn all the time to absorb saliva. Oral intake of foods was not even considered to be a possibility.

Goals

Thomas and I agreed on the following treatment goals.

Long-Term Goal
- To remove the nasogastric tube and eat and drink orally

Short-Term Goals
- To alleviate fear, inspire confidence in me and my therapeutic approach, and establish a comfort zone for therapy exercises
- To introduce tactile stimuli within the oral area
- To improve lip and jaw closure
- To diminish or extinguish drooling
- To facilitate tongue and jaw movements for mastication
- To encourage speech

INTERVENTION

All visits with Thomas were 1–2 weeks apart with phone consultations with the nurses on duty in between those visits. These wonderful nurses were supportive of Thomas at all times. The nurses and I maintained contact with the primary care physician.

SECOND VISIT (2 WEEKS LATER)

Thomas was slowly gaining confidence in me and allowed me to feed him a drop of thin applesauce and a tiny drop of nectar juice (a thick liquid) from a spoon. Thomas and I then worked out a home program together. We thoroughly discussed the prescribed procedures in order to decrease his fear. The nursing staff was present to observe, question, and assist with the procedures.

Home Program	Rationale
Practice the preparatory spoon technique. As Thomas is quite fearful, he prefers that the nurse place the empty teaspoon on top of his tongue. The nurse slides an uncoated, *nonplastic*, empty teaspoon at a 45 degree angle over the lower lip with a light touch. The bowl of the spoon then is rested flat on top of the tongue with firm but gentle pressure applied for 2 seconds. The spoon is withdrawn with a slight downward movement. This will be done three times daily (Figure 5).	This exercise helps Thomas adjust to tactile input in preparation for actual food. The withdrawal position encourages lip closure on the spoon.

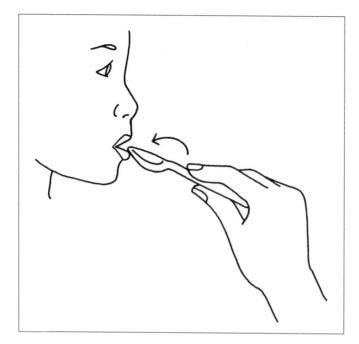

Figure 5
Lip-closure technique using a spoon.

Home Program	Rationale
Remember to maintain a centered head position with only slight flexion in order to prevent an upward movement of the jaw (Figure 6).	Thomas tends to thrust his chin forward in an exaggerated fashion for swallowing. It is important to maintain a slightly flexed and centered head position while swallowing in order to prevent coughing or discomfort.
Perform the saliva swallowing exercise three times a day, three to five repetitions each time. A swallow is performed with an upright, slightly flexed, and centered head position with the tip of the tongue pressed upward on the hard palate.	Thomas needs to be more aware of the positioning of his tongue and the swallowing of his saliva.

THIRD VISIT (1 WEEK LATER)

Thomas has done well with his exercises. I am very pleased that he now wishes to try the swallow exercise with food.

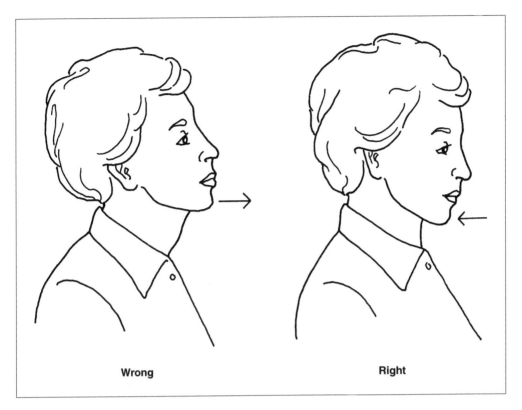

Wrong

Right

Figure 6
Examples of correct and incorrect chin-tuck positions.

Home Program	Rationale
Perform the lip-shaking exercise with the top lip only. This will be repeated twice three times a day before the spoon exercise. Thomas will use his thumb and index finger to gently but firmly shake the top lip, moving one corner down and toward the center, then moving the center of the lip down, and finally moving the opposite lip corner down toward the center. This creates a somewhat "pursed" appearance of the lip. Each area will be wiggled three times (Figure 7).	This exercise helps develop lip closure so Thomas can later close his lips on the spoon and cup. Improving lip closure also diminishes drooling. Tactile defensiveness should also decrease. Concentrating on one lip at a time reduces confusion and makes learning easier.

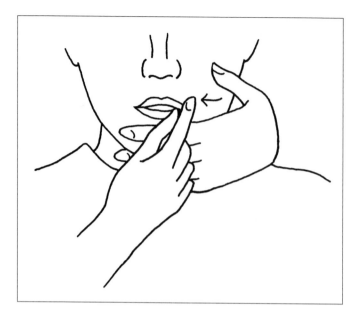

Figure 7
Lip-closure technique using lip shaking.

Home Program	Rationale
Stabilize elbows on a table (or lap tray) and use one hand (left) to place the middle finger under the chin with the index finger parallel to and just below the lower lip. The thumb is held parallel to the face and away from the eye (Figure 8).	This independent head and jaw stabilization posture keeps the chin *tucked in* and prevents the jaw from jutting out. This technique is helpful for many independent patients who tend to swallow with abnormal head positioning, jaw opening, and an open mouth.
Continue using the spoon technique (with ¼ teaspoon of nectar juice or runny applesauce) while maintaining the independent head and jaw control position. This exercise should follow the lip-shaking exercise. Thomas may repeat this technique as long as he is comfortable doing so.	Using a thickened liquid is often the best way to introduce oral intake. It is important to use only ¼ of a teaspoon or less at the beginning. Hopefully, the lip-shaking and spoon technique exercises, therapy and practicum, will encourage lip-closure movements. Thomas still prefers for the nurse to place the spoon for him.

FOURTH VISIT (2 WEEKS LATER)

Thomas is unhappy that he still has little feeling in his tongue and top lip. I reassure him that the feeling will come with time and remind him that he cannot expect too

Figure 8
Use of the controlled hand position for independent head and jaw stabilization.

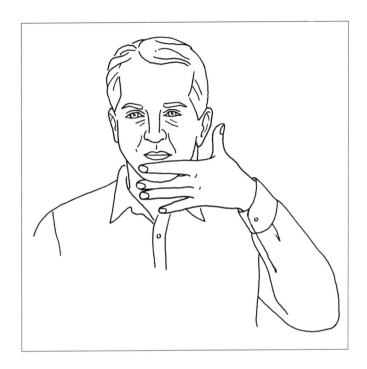

much after only three visits. He continues to have problems with drooling. However, he is working hard to make positive changes by performing his therapeutic exercises regularly. We continue to engage in extensive conversation—Thomas writes on the pad he uses for communication and I answer. I feel confident that we have established a comfort zone in our relationship. The nursing staff asks many questions and is engaged in the entire process. Together, we continue to make progress.

Home Program	Rationale
Continue the lip shaking before performing the spoon exercise.	Lip shaking needs to be maintained to stimulate the muscles. Following this manual exercise with the practicum (the spoon technique) generally produces good results. Patients can usually see and feel results rather quickly with the combination of these exercises.
Continue the spoon technique using ¼ teaspoon of blended, canned pudding (Thomas's choice of food).	Thomas now wants to try a therapeutic exercise independently—a big step for him. He is confident that he will not have any coughing accidents. Also, one of our short-term goals has been met—tactile defensiveness within the oral

Home Program	Rationale
	area appears to have disappeared. (Great.)
Attempt sipping a tiny amount of thinned pudding or nectar from a cup with independent head and jaw control. I recommend placing the cup on the lip with slight pressure and sipping slowly. If cup drinking produces stress, the exercise should be discontinued for the present time.	Thomas wishes to try the cup. I feel certain he will sip as suggested. It is important to Thomas's morale to move on to new skills.
Remember the chin tuck head position.	Thomas wishes to stop using the independent head and jaw control position with the spoon, so I ask him to concentrate on awareness of head position.
Encourage Thomas to practice the selected words and sounds assigned by his speech therapist.	The nursing staff and I consistently encourage Thomas to follow through on his speech therapy exercises. He prefers not to try and continues to write reams of notes to me.

FIFTH VISIT (1 WEEK LATER)

Thomas now performs two or more consecutive, but abnormal, open-mouth swallows with each ¼ teaspoon of pudding. He wishes to increase his food intake and is very pleased with and encouraged by his progress. He needs to be reminded to hold his head in the centered position with only slight flexion for the swallows. Thomas happily states that he now has "slight feeling" in his top lip. This sensation increases his ability to sip from a cup or spoon. Thomas talks more and more about his anger at being tied down by all of his physical problems. He also talks enthusiastically about his love for music and composing. He is anxious to return to the stage.

Home Program	Rationale
Continue home program outlined in the fourth visit.	This will ensure that Thomas continues his progress toward meeting his goals. All of these exercises help diminish drooling and develop normal jaw and lip closure, the ability to orally intake nutritious foods, improve lip closure on the cup and spoon, and encourage normal swallowing.

SIXTH VISIT (1 WEEK LATER)

Thomas is now swallowing 10¼ teaspoons of his favored pudding consecutively. Increased oral intake has begun! Thomas is very pleased. We continue discussion (with Thomas using his writing pad) before and after each suggestion I make. Thomas is very alert and aware and, as always, eager to state his thoughts about everything. He continues to feed himself and states he has both good and bad days. His gag reflex now appears normal. Some drooling continues; therefore, it is necessary to again use independent head and jaw control when eating or drinking.

Home Program	Rationale
Use independent head and jaw control when eating or drinking.	This will reinforce correct head positioning and decrease drooling.
Practice the lip-shaking exercise with both the top and bottom lips. The bottom lip is wiggled upward and toward the center. Top lip exercises should continue as described in the third visit.	Continuing these exercises will help develop bilabial lip closure.
Continue the spoon and cup exercise following the lip-shaking exercise. Pudding or nectar may be used. After the thick nectar can be comfortably and safely swallowed, try ¼ teaspoon of water or broth.	A thickened liquid is easier to handle initially because it moves slowly through the pharynx, decreasing the risk of aspiration.
Begin practicing the normal coordinated swallow. Maintain a centered head position with head and jaw control. Saliva swallows will be practiced with the mouth *closed* one to two times, three times a day. (See *second visit.*) If this is done comfortably, a tiny swallow may be attempted with nectar or water (Thomas's choice).	The automatic coordinated swallow is usually difficult for a patient. The cognitive swallow must be learned before the automatic swallow. (We are aware of the cognitive swallow. We are not aware of the automatic swallow.)

SEVENTH VISIT (1 WEEK LATER)

Thomas enjoys our conversations because they help answer his numerous questions and relieve his occasional concerns. Even though progress is evident, a bit of mucus or coughing interferes occasionally with his daily routine. Thomas now feels more comfortable and is able to deal with this problem without panic by correcting his head position. Suctioning is rarely needed—another goal has been reached! As always, I review the exercises with Thomas during the visit. The coordinated swallow was attempted with the cup and Thomas now states that he has increased feeling in his mouth. The nurses report that Thomas now consumes 80% of an 8-oz cup of liquid in one day using a combination of coordinated and uncoordinated swallows. Drooling is greatly diminished. Thomas is moving ahead much faster than I had anticipated. I am also told that he is walking about (within his room) more than he had been doing previously.

Thomas's ability to repeat successful coordinated and uncoordinated swallows with juice, water, and pudding varies. One day he may have to rest after five swallows and the next day he will perform 20 swallows without rest. He alternates between using the spoon and the cup. The amount of drooling varies from day to day and does not appear to be related to the type of oral intake.

Home Program	Rationale
Continue lip-shaking exercises with both the top and bottom lip three times a day followed by the cup exercise.	Continue integration of lip-closure skills.
Drink water, broth, or Sustacal (recommended by the nurses) from a cup. I suggest maintaining the cup on the lip for a few seconds after the liquid is sipped into the mouth.	This drinking will increase oral intake of liquids and help Thomas practice lip closure. Slight pressure on the lip appears to help Thomas maintain closed lips in preparation for the normal coordinated swallow.
Increase oral intake using the spoon or cup and small amounts of applesauce with Sustacal. This is done two to three times daily.	The nursing staff had suggested this mixture to increase the nutritional value of oral intake.
Practice coordinated swallows with water or broth.	Thomas wishes to continue integrative, coordinated swallows with the thin liquid. He feels comfortable with his ability to swallow thickened liquids.
Maintain independent head and jaw control.	Thomas needs to continue practicing correct head positioning.

EIGHTH VISIT (2 WEEKS LATER)

Thomas is anxious to have the nasogastric tube removed. He is eating a good quantity of the applesauce and Sustacal mixture and the nurses have reduced the frequency of tube feedings by 50%. He is now less confined and enthusiastic and beaming. Although I am very pleased with his progress, I do not think that Thomas should have the tube removed at this time because he occasionally has mucus build up and is only in the beginning stage of success with the coordinated swallow. Drooling continues to be erratic and we have not even begun to work on chewing skills. Thomas rather reluctantly agrees to continue therapy and not remove the nasogastric tube.

Home Program	Rationale
Continue lip-shaking exercise three times a day.	This will maintain Thomas's lip closure skills.
Incorporate smooth food into the practice of the coordinated swallow with independent head and jaw control. Begin with saliva swallows and move on to the mixture of applesauce and Sustacal (three swallows, three times a day).	Thomas states that he is now ready and eager to begin normal swallows with smooth foods.

NINTH VISIT (2 WEEKS LATER)

The nurses report that Sustacal may have been causing the excess mucus production. We substitute applesauce diluted with water and the problem appears to be alleviated. Thomas is now drinking warm tea and cranberry juice and making his own foods, including "instant breakfast" drinks and milk shakes with papaya, banana, and ice milk. He is experimenting with additional blended combinations. His coordinated swallow is progressing well. When fatigued, Thomas alternates with the saliva-swallowing exercise and continues performing the lip-shaking exercise before eating. Head control is now almost perfect without reminders or independent head and jaw stabilization. Drooling is diminished but still occurs at times.

Thomas is feeling very optimistic and cheerful. He even invited me into his music studio (located next to his bedroom) so that he could play a couple of his compositions on the piano for me.

Home Program	Rationale
Practice the following tongue movements: (1) raise the tongue upward as if to touch the upper lip and (2) attempt to move the tongue about 1/16 in. to the right of the center of the top lip. If this is successful, the tongue may be moved a bit further and the exercise repeated on the left side. This exercise should be done twice daily for 1–2 minutes.	These exercises will increase and improve the tongue's range of motion vertically and laterally in preparation for chewing textured foods.

Home Program	Rationale
Practice coordinated saliva swallows. If relaxed, try coordinated swallows with a blended food mixture of any desired thickness.	Saliva swallows are easy, safe, and comforting. Thomas is eager to move on.

TENTH VISIT (2 WEEKS LATER)

Thomas has decided against my wishes that he will ask his physician to remove the nasogastric tube immediately. He thinks it is time for him to "move back into life's stream." His coordinated swallows are more consistent at this time and he tells me he does "not care to learn how to chew." He knows he can continue to live well on a blended diet and is satisfied with that outcome. Thomas realizes that he will have to be careful to drink small amounts of liquid slowly and leave the cup on his lip for a few seconds before withdrawing to swallow to prevent spills. He also will carry numerous handkerchiefs and tissues with him to wipe up the occasional excess saliva. None of these precautions appears to be distressing to Thomas. He looks forward to conducting and composing and "living in the real world again."

Thomas began blending his own foods, went back to work, and was happy. He no longer required nursing care. I received a beautiful letter from him a few weeks later thanking me for "rescuing" him and allowing him to return to the world he loved—composing and conducting. I enjoy listening to his music on television and radio.

CONCLUSION

Two years after I stopped working with Thomas I read in the newspaper that he had died of amyotrophic lateral sclerosis (ALS) (Lou Gehrig's disease). In the early 1980s, little was known of ALS and, therefore, Thomas went undiagnosed until shortly before his death. Neuromuscular symptoms were evident at the time of treatment, including progressive muscle weakness, tongue and jaw involvement, and lack of speech. We now understand that the myelin sheath is destroyed or replaced by scar tissue, and nerve impulses become distorted or blocked in ALS patients. This progressive degeneration causes extensive muscle weakness and atrophy until the patient becomes unable to take care of his or her physical needs. Respiratory problems develop and total nursing care may be required.

I am extremely gratified that Thomas was able to live comfortably and as he wished for as long as possible. I am indebted to his nursing staff for their constant support and cooperation. They were there for Thomas all of the time, encouraged each new endeavor, and helped me in every way with Thomas's therapy. Therefore, I was able to treat him symptomatically and functionally in a supportive fashion.

Length of intervention: 3 months, 10 visits.

The Case of
The Mysterious
Ailment:
Dysautonomia

DESCRIPTION AND PRESENTING PROBLEM

Allan was 4 years old when his mother brought him to see me. She was extremely anxious, visibly shaken, and determined to engage my services. She had searched for treatment for Allan's feeding problems for many months and it seemed to her as if there were no therapists that could help them. Allan had been diagnosed with dysautonomia, and although conferences and studies of the disorder were going on and outstanding specialists from all over the world were researching it, in 1972 few therapists knew of or had treated dysautonomia. It seemed to Allan's family that there was no one in California who could treat him. I had never even heard of this disorder. Treating Allan promised to be a challenge.

Dysautonomia is a disorder of the autonomic nervous system. The condition is hereditary and predominantly affects Jews from Northern Europe. It was first diagnosed by the physicians Riley and Day in 1949. Difficulty breathing, poor or absent sucking and swallowing skills, absent taste buds, inability to produce tears, unstable blood pressure, uncontrollable vomiting, pneumonia, indifference to pain, and hypersensitivity to touch are a few of the physical problems these patients have. These overwhelming physical problems cause psychological and social problems for the patient and his or her family. The family endures stress and constant fear every day. Affected children are frequently very intelligent and could do exceedingly well in mainstream society if they did not have severe physical disabilities. Even though Allan was ambulatory, Allan's mother stated that it was impossible for him to participate in activities with other children because of his frequent hospitalizations.

FIRST VISIT

The pre-speech, oral-motor feeding evaluation indicated the following dysfunctions.

Dysfunction	Explanation
Absence of sucking motions	A disorder of the autonomic system
Uncoordinated, abnormal, open-mouth swallowing	Inadequate oral-motor control

Dysfunction	Explanation
Open mouth/oral breathing	The breathing and swallowing pattern is uncoordinated.
Absence of lip closure	Decreased muscle control inhibits Allan's ability to close his lips on the spoon and cup.
A protruding, pointed tongue that thrusts forward frequently	Tongue movements are abnormal due to lack of oral-motor control.
Drooling	Drooling is a result of an open mouth, abnormal swallows, and decreased muscle control.
No oral intake (tube feeding only)	When he was 3 years old, Allan had a severe case of pneumonia and ceased all oral intake.
Sensory defensiveness, especially around the head, upper torso and mouth	Allan's parents report that he became hypersensitive to touch after the case of pneumonia.
Vomiting episodes for no obvious reason	These are characteristic of dysautonomia in some patients.
Absence of speech	Allan is a bright and aware child whose diminished oral-motor control contributes to his inability to produce intelligible speech. He communicates by grunting and pointing.
Rejection of any oral intake	This rejection is common among people who are tube fed and sensory defensive within the mouth.
Ataxic gait, poor balance in upper and lower extremities, and alternating periods of hyperactivity and hypoactivity.	These problems are all characteristic of Allan's dysautonomia.

I asked Allan's mother to alert me immediately if she noticed any physical problems developing during our visits. Because Allan was my first patient with dysautonomia, I thought I might not recognize subtle signs of distress. I informed Allan's parents that I would discuss my work with Allan's primary care physician. I contacted many speech-language pathologists, physical therapists, and occupational therapists, hoping to talk to someone who had worked with patients with dysautonomia. None of them had, but they offered their support for my work with Allan.

Goals

Allan's mother and I agreed on the following treatment goals for Allan.

Long-Term Goals

- To end tube feedings
- To eat and drink orally
- To encourage chewing skills
- To encourage normal breathing and swallowing patterns
- To encourage speech

Short-Term Goals

- To establish rapport between Allan, his mother, and me
- To decrease sensory defensiveness
- To eliminate vomiting
- To introduce oral intake of foods
- To stop tongue thrusting
- To encourage bilabial lip closure

INTERVENTION

Therapy sessions took place either in my office or in Allan's home. Visits in the home were frequently necessary because Allan had pneumonia, medication problems, posthospitalization trauma, and other illnesses. It was easier for mother and Allan if I came to their home on occasion. Visits were frequently many weeks apart; therefore, I made sure that Allan felt comfortable with me at each visit by playing and "talking" with him before we worked on therapeutic exercises. I also tried to talk privately before each session with Allan's mother about her anxiety, fears, and hopes as well as about Allan and his needs. At each visit, as is my custom, I observed her feeding Allan his preferred food snacks, which I requested she bring. I also fed Allan myself before we wrote the home program together.

SECOND VISIT (1 WEEK LATER)

Allan was hyperactive today, but we were able to play together with toys that he handled very well. I even received a spontaneous gentle hug and a light kiss on my hand. Drooling was not excessive even though Allan's tongue protruded frequently and his mouth was always open. His mother told me that Allan could not drink any liquids because of the congestion and coughing that resulted. She has attempted to feed him some smooth foods, however. I can, therefore, begin working with the spoon and oral intake of foods immediately.

Home Program	Rationale
Perform sensory play with a thin (transparent) scarf on top of the face, mouth games to encourage more sounds, hugging games, and peek-a-boo with Allan's hands on his face. Rub the entire body (excluding the face) with a nubby towel using a brisk, firm, but gentle up-and-down rubbing motion. Begin with the lower extremities and move up to the torso, arms, and shoulders. Repeat this exercise as often as possible each day.	Sensory play and brisk, firm rubbing of the body help to decrease sensory defensiveness. A light touch usually causes a negative response; a firm touch appears to inhibit discomfort. Mouth games encourage improved communication and allow tactile stimulation around the oral area. Because the mouth is the most sensitive area, I do not rub the face until the patient accepts a fair amount of stimulation on the body.
Feed ¼ teaspoon of pudding one to two times daily if the food is accepted comfortably.	A smooth, preferred food is a good way to begin oral intake. Tiny amounts are used to prevent coughing, choking, or aspiration. A slightly thickened texture is easier to handle because it moves slowly through the pharynx, decreasing the risk of aspiration.
Feed ¼ teaspoon of a smooth, thinned chili one to two times daily if the food is accepted comfortably.	A strong flavor is appropriate because of Allan's apparent diminished taste buds. His mother emphatically insisted we try adding chili.

THIRD VISIT (4 WEEKS LATER)

Allan's mother reports that he "loved the chili and did not vomit." She decided to add crushed bacon bits, which Allan loved. Mother is impatient and I think she will continue to try new foods on her own. My assessment indicates that Allan is not quite ready for textured food such as bacon bits. I hesitate to push him too far and too fast. However, mothers frequently are able to assess their children's abilities as well as, if not better than, a professional. Nonetheless, a therapist must be aware of frustrations and dangers that may occur without the caregiver noticing. Fear of food, rejection, coughing, choking, and aspiration could all jeopardize Allan's treatment and safety.

Home Program	Rationale
Apply firm but gentle pressure with an uncoated, nonplastic,	The uncoated spoon provides sensory input. The slight tea-

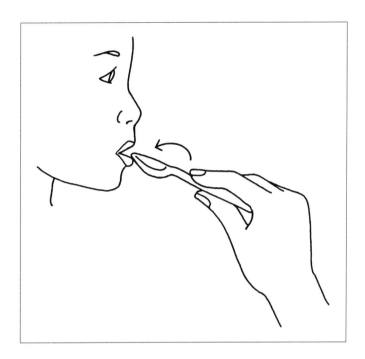

Figure 9
Lip-closure technique using a spoon.

Home Program	Rationale
shallow teaspoon with ¼ teaspoon of smooth pudding halfway back on the tongue. The spoon should be positioned at a 45-degree angle as it slides in with a light touch on the lower lip. The bowl of the spoon needs to rest flat on top of the tongue. Pressure should be maintained for approximately 2 seconds. This exercise should be done one to two times, twice daily (Figure 9).	spoon pressure increases the sensory input and frequently helps diminish tongue thrust. The bowl of the spoon should be shallow so that it encourages good lip closure. I have found it more efficient to place the index finger on top of the spoon handle.
Use applesauce or any strained food with bacon bits (mother's preference) for oral intake (without applying spoon pressure) for two to three bites three times a day.	For now, spoon pressure should not be used with the added food texture. Introducing one new exercise at a time is sufficient to encourage progress. Because Allan does "munch" his foods, limited texture is safe at this time.
Continue sensory games.	Maintenance of sensory input exercises should continue to

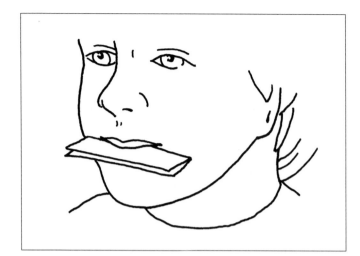

Figure 10
Lip-closure technique using aluminum foil.

Home Program	Rationale
	decrease sensitivity. These exercises will eventually include rubbing on the face.
Attempt to hold a folded piece of aluminum foil between closed lips for as long as possible (Figure 10).	This exercise encourages bilabial lip closure and the normal coordinated swallow. The foil is an excellent treatment material because it does not stick to the lips and is a pleasing material for patients of all ages. Allan appeared eager to try this activity.

FOURTH VISIT (4 WEEKS LATER)

I have not seen Allan for a month due to his respiratory illness. His mother tells me that in addition to abnormal tongue thrust, Allan is purposely pushing his tongue forward. I explained that because these movements appear to be done purposely and with playful intent we should just ignore them for now. Therapy has continued quite well at home. Mother and I are both very pleased and Allan appears content.

Home Program	Rationale
Continue sensory input using towel on the body. Begin rubbing the face also. A nubby towel may be used occasionally during the day to wipe face and hands. Play with modeling clay,	These activities maintain sensory input. Because Allan rarely objects to sensory input on his body, rubbing on the face and around the mouth can now be added. The games

Figure 11
Lip-closure technique using a spoon.

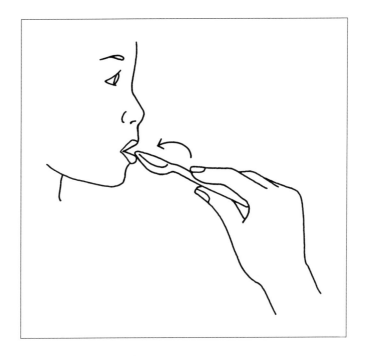

Home Program	Rationale
ice cubes, and sand (dry, damp, or wet) to increase sensory input.	provide experience with additional textures and consistencies. Modeling clay should be used first because it has a consistent texture. Dry sand is smooth but pebbly. Adding varying amounts of water creates slightly different textures and weights. Exposure to these different textures helps decrease Allan's hypersensitivity.
Continue applying spoon pressure (with pudding) on the tongue for three to five bites as often as Allan will permit.	Because Allan has accepted this exercise, the number of times it is performed is increased.
Use the spoon to encourage lip closure. Lightly press the spoon *downward* while slowly withdrawing it. Perform this exercise during snack and meal times (Figure 11).	This exercise encourages lip closure on the spoon and retraction of the tongue.
Clean gums with fine gauze or with a baby toothbrush twice daily for a few minutes.	Now that Allan accepts tactile input within his mouth, his mother will be able to improve his dental hygiene.

Home Program	Rationale
Discontinue the aluminum foil game for now.	This game was providing too much input for Allan and he resisted the activity.

FIFTH VISIT (2 WEEKS LATER)

Allan's mother, delighted with his progress, continues to push ahead faster than I would like. When Allan rejects her attempts, however, she understands that she must slow down and accept his rate of progress. Because Allan is happily accepting a few spoons of food, I suggested that we now have him eat with other people. Allan has always been fed separately from others and he needs to join his family and other children whenever possible.

Home Program	Rationale
Continue all therapeutic exercises assigned in the third and fourth visit.	Allan appears to happily accept all these exercises and continuation will promote maintenance and skill integration.
Begin performing the graham cracker exercise with head and jaw control at the beginning of a meal once or twice only. If head and jaw control is accepted, the exercise may be repeated in the middle of the meal once or twice only. This exercise should be performed with the caregiver at the patient's side with the nondominant hand coming around the patient's body so that fingers extend to cup the chin without squeezing. The index finger should remain stationary under the lower lip. The third finger is placed under the chin with the thumb held away from the face and eyes. The other hand places a small piece of graham cracker between the molars on one side of the mouth. When the cracker is either melted or chewed and swallowed, a piece of similar size is placed on the opposite side of the mouth. Beginning lateral	Head and jaw control must be used to maintain *centering* of the head to encourage tongue lateralization for chewing. However, it is important that this control is gentle. Demonstrating the position on the caregiver relieves tension and concern about the position looking like a head lock. Performing this exercise too frequently may discourage oral intake. Snack time is an excellent time to introduce this activity.

Figure 12
Graham cracker exercise to encourage chewing movements.

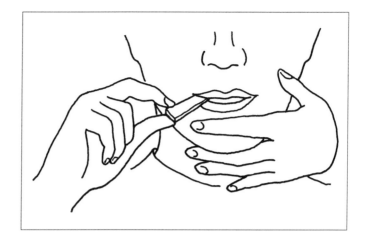

Home Program	Rationale
tongue and jaw movements should be observed (Figure 12).	
Add new textured foods such as large-curd cottage cheese, mushy corn flakes, mushy egg salad, and scrambled eggs.	These textures can be added because of Allan's acceptance and more forceful munching.
Center the head and hold an ice cream cone to each side of the mouth. This should be done twice daily, for two to three licks on each side.	This tongue lateralization exercise is fun and tasty.

SIXTH VISIT (4 WEEKS LATER)

Allan is now consuming a fair amount of food orally. I think he is ready to substitute oral feeding for one of his regular tube feedings. He has also happily accepted the head and jaw control for a few minutes. Mother is very pleased that Allan is enjoying his new foods and no longer vomits. I suggest that Allan try using a straw to drink small amounts of liquid. Mother, however, does not think that Allan is ready for oral liquid intake.

Home Program	Rationale
Consult with a nutritionist.	The nutritionist can provide assistance planning nutritious, well-balanced meals.
Continue applying pressure on the tongue with a spoon but with head and jaw control. (See	Using head and jaw control with the spoon pressure and simultaneous slight head flex-

Home Program	Rationale
fifth visit.) Perform this exercise twice at each meal and snack period or as often as Allan will accept it.	ion will greatly increase the potential for lip closure.
Place a raspberry seed (from jam) or a dab of honey on the top lip. The tongue should be used to reach upward to the center of the lips to capture the seed. If the exercise is successful, the seed (or honey) will move $\frac{1}{16}$ in. to one side, then $\frac{1}{16}$ in. to the other side until the seed and tongue touch the corners of the lips.	This exercise increases tongue movements and is fun.
Discontinue the sensory games. Continue towel rubbing and hugging at bath time.	Because Allan is comfortable with sensory input, the games can be discontinued. Sensory input should be maintained, however, with towel rubbing and hugging.
Encourage play with developmental toys.	Toys and games should help Allan develop fine motor coordination while having fun. Allan needs toys that are more challenging and stimulating than those he currently has.
Encourage use of words instead of pointing or grunting to indicate a desired object.	Allan has good beginning tongue, lip, and jaw movements and needs encouragement to attempt communication with speech.

SEVENTH VISIT (4 WEEKS LATER)

Allan now demonstrates minimal lateralization of the tongue and horizontal jaw movements, indicating that his chewing ability is developing. The nutritionist suggested the following foods that Allan is now eating: mashed banana with milk powder, coarsely blended fruit cocktail, hot cereal with milk powder, soft scrambled eggs, spaghetti rings, chili, tuna, egg or mashed chicken salad with mayonnaise and garlic salt, and rice. It is no longer necessary to limit Allan to smooth foods—his ability to move his lips, tongue, and jaws is improving. We can now eliminate another tube feeding.

Exercises will now emphasize improving tongue and jaw movements for chewing skills, lip closure, and the coordinated swallow. Occasional tongue protrusion continues. Improving lip closure and tongue lateralization should decrease this problem. Drooling is also decreasing for the same reasons and Allan no longer has to wear a bib to protect his clothing. He now babbles, points to communicate rather than grunting, and uses a few words!

Home Program	Rationale
Consult with a speech-language pathologist.	Allan's prespeech skills are improving and additional therapy should improve Allan's communication skills.
Continue practicing the spoon exercise with head and jaw control. Increase the number of times to Allan's comfort level.	This exercise will continue to improve lip closure, decrease tongue thrusting, and diminish drooling.
Play straw blowing games.	These games stimulate lip-pursing movements.
Discontinue raspberry-seed game.	Allan did not wish to do this activity.
Try the aluminum foil game again once or twice daily.	This can be a fun game to increase lip closure time for the acquisition of the coordinated swallow. A group of children (or family) can be challenged to see who can hold the foil between the lips the longest time. Allan now appears ready to try this activity.

EIGHTH VISIT (4 WEEKS LATER)

Allan's family has been pressuring him to eat more. This has caused differences of opinion between his mother and me. Discussing these differences helps a bit, but mother is eager to be free of the burden of tube feedings. She is now anxious to survey appropriate school situations, especially because drooling and tongue protrusion are rare.

Home Program	Rationale
Decrease the pressure on Allan to eat more.	Allan needs rewards for any amount of food he consumes, including hugs and loving remarks.
Eat bran buds soaked for 15–20 minutes in nonfat milk with 1 tablespoon of molasses.	I have used this recipe, which was given to me by a nutritionist, for many patients of all ages to decrease constipation.

Home Program	Rationale
Increase the amount of spices added to foods.	This should increase Allan's desire to eat and enjoyment of his foods.
Blend food less and encourage chewing of foods such as crisped-rice cereals and wide cheese puffs. Sweets should not be eaten at this time.	Chewing these foods will help develop better tongue and jaw movement skills. Sweets should be avoided so that healthy food is eaten first.
Continue to ask Allan to use words to indicate his desire for a particular object. Reward all attempts with verbal reinforcement or hugs.	This exercise is done in conjunction with the speech-language pathologist.
Mother has chosen to eliminate another tube feeding (with nutritionist's approval). Two of four tube feedings have now been eliminated. Add extra liquids to foods to compensate for the fact that Allan still does not drink liquids.	Allan is eating enough oral foods to allow the decrease in tube feedings.
Continue exercises assigned at the last visit.	These exercises will ensure continued improvement and skill integration.

CONCLUSION

During 5½ months of therapy, Allan was hospitalized frequently between our visits. However, he still was able to make satisfactory progress toward meeting treatment goals. Sensory defensiveness and tongue protrusion stopped, oral intake improved significantly, and he was close to achieving excellent chewing skills with varying textures of food. Allan's mother chose at this time to discontinue feeding therapy and to stop using any tube feedings. She did not consult with Allan's primary care physician, however. She thought that with the assistance of the nutritionist she would be able to maintain a healthy diet for Allan. Therefore, she enrolled Allan in an appropriate school setting. She hoped that he would learn to socialize with children of his own age. She was at last free to live a more normal life. Life was rapidly changing for Allan and his family.

I thought much work still needed to be done. We had attained many of our initial goals, but reaching more would better ensure Allan's comfort, oral-motor competence, and pleasure. His rotary chewing skills were just beginning to develop. Lip closure and the coordinated swallow were still not constant and Allan was continuing to receive all of his liquids in his foods. Allan could, however, manage nicely (and safely) in an appropriate school setting. However, the family thought Allan was progressing well and I could no longer anticipate they would follow through with the home program. Therefore, Allan's feeding therapy ended.

Allan's mother kept in touch by phone for 1 year. Allan and his family were enjoying their increased freedom, and I was happy for all of them. They had even taken Allan to McDonald's!

Approximately 2 years later, I learned that Allan had died during an episode of pneumonia.

Length of intervention: 5.5 months, 8 visits

The Case of the Noisy Swallower: Cerebral Palsy with Articulation Problems

DESCRIPTION AND PRESENTING PROBLEM

Nancy, an attractive 15½ year old, walked into my office with a limping gait. She told me that she had cerebral palsy and that she was bothered more by her noisy swallowing than her limp. "My swallow is so noisy that people always know when I'm in a room before they even see me," she said. She wanted to socialize with her friends without embarrassment. She was also taking driving lessons to be more independent.

Nancy had no other medical problems. She was able to eat nutritious meals. She did have occasional difficulties eating highly textured foods and minor coughing episodes. She did not have any drooling problems. Previous occupational and physical therapy sessions had not addressed the problems of coughing, loud swallows, or slightly impaired speech.

FIRST VISIT

The pre-speech oral-motor feeding evaluation indicated the following dysfunctions.

Dysfunction	Explanation
Occasional abnormal, loud, uncoordinated swallows	Nancy swallows food and liquid using an open-mouth swallow because of poor oral-motor control caused by neurologic dysfunction. I do not know what causes the loud swallowing.
Mixed oral and nasal breathing	A combination of normal swallows (closed mouth) and abnormal swallows (open mouth)
Limited range, mobility, and cupping of the tongue	Decreased muscle tone and oral-motor control

Dysfunction	Explanation
Some large, unchewed pieces of food are swallowed. Occasional small coughs occur, but no gagging or aspiration is noted.	Nancy has limited lateral and vertical movements of the tongue and jaw. She has not acquired rotation and mature chewing movements because of decreased muscle tone and poor oral-motor control.
Frequent swallowing after each bite, usually with slight hyperextension of the head and occasional small coughs. Foods such as hamburger and apple tend to dissipate throughout her mouth. Nancy explains that she "swallows a lot to get rid of the food spread around in my mouth."	Because Nancy has difficulty forming and preparing a food bolus with her tongue, she chews longer than normal before each swallow. Occasionally, small particles of food spill down into the trachea when she swallows with her head in hyperextension. This hyperextension makes swallowing easier but results in coughing.
Slight articulation difficulties	Chewing, swallowing, and speech muscles are the same; decreased muscle tone and control, therefore, also affects Nancy's speech.

Goals

Nancy and I agreed on the following treatment goals.

Long-Term Goals

- To eliminate excess swallowing
- To diminish the exceedingly loud sounds
- To improve chewing skills
- To acquire normal, closed-mouth, coordinated breathing and swallowing patterns
- To improve speech

Short-Term Goals

- To develop a normal head position for swallowing
- To learn improved tongue and jaw movements for chewing skills
- To decrease the number of excess swallows

INTERVENTION

Nancy brought samples of her preferred foods (both heavily textured and smooth) to all visits so I could observe her skills. Our communication during these sessions was easygoing and comfortable. Her mother, who drove her to therapy sessions, was often included in these conversations.

SECOND VISIT (1 WEEK LATER)

Nancy and her mother arrived at my office eager to begin therapy, which they both hoped would end Nancy's loud swallowing. I carefully observed Nancy eating her own lunch while we talked about Nancy's activities in school. This diverted attention from the eating process. We agreed on the following home program of exercises.

Home Program	Rationale
Practice three to four saliva swallows three times per day. Place the tip of the tongue on the hard palate for each swallow.	One of the first steps Nancy needs to learn in preparation for the normal, coordinated swallow is correct placement of the tongue for swallowing. It is acceptable for Nancy to continue swallowing with an open mouth *at this time.*
Remember to swallow smooth food with the head slightly flexed for two swallows three times per day.	Because Nancy does swallow occasionally with head flexion, she may only need written reminders (e.g., written notes posted in her room and kitchen).

THIRD VISIT (1 WEEK LATER)

Nancy did her exercises every day and demonstrates good cognitive control of her tongue movements. She has found that the exercises require concentration and significant effort, particularly to maintain correct head position.

Home Program	Rationale
Continue practicing the saliva swallows.	Nancy should continue this exercise until she is comfortable with it.
Thin the highly textured foods at home and take smaller bites.	This is a preventive method to reduce the amount of food in the mouth so that coughing episodes decrease. This should also encourage cupping movements of the tongue and make it easier for Nancy to chew bites more thoroughly before

	swallowing (less food in the mouth makes it easier for the tongue to move about).

FOURTH VISIT (1 WEEK LATER)

Nancy is less enthusiastic today. "Therapy is not as much fun as I thought—it's hard work," she says. Our communication is excellent, however, and we talk about her frustrations. I remind her that therapy can be tedious and lengthy but generally has very positive results. As always, we thoroughly discuss and agree on the home program for next week.

Home Program	Rationale
Continue saliva swallows with cognitive awareness of the tongue position (three times daily for three to four swallows each time).	Nancy should continue to integrate her skills. Her tongue movement begins to improve.
Perform swallows with a drop of plain yogurt (three times daily for three swallows each time before school, after school, and in the evenings).	A drop of smooth food can be safely introduced because Nancy is now able to maintain a slightly flexed head position for swallowing.
Continue thinning textured foods and taking smaller bites.	Because it is too soon to begin another new exercise, Nancy should continue using these preventive methods.

FIFTH VISIT (2 WEEKS LATER)

It has been 2 weeks since Nancy's last visit because she had a cold. She is pleased with therapy results and anxious to move ahead at a faster rate. This is a request made by many of my patients.

Home Program	Rationale
Begin the quick swallow exercise with a drop of plain, thinned yogurt (three times daily for two to four swallows each time). The container of yogurt is positioned just beneath the lower lip and kept there for the entire exercise. The spoon	Tongue movement is improving as Nancy becomes more comfortable. She is also improving her ability to swallow normally with a substance in her mouth. It is easier for her to swallow several times with a small amount of food

Figure 13
Quick swallow exercise to facilitate normal swallowing time

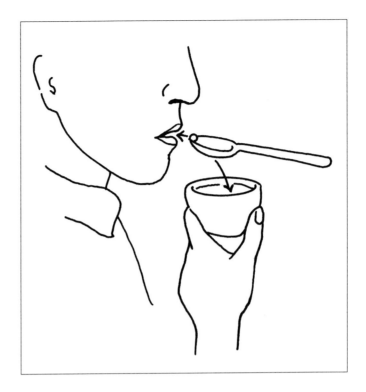

Home Program	Rationale
should only touch the yogurt and then be placed quickly into the mouth for the swallow. This process should be done as quickly as is comfortable (Figure 13).	than swallow a large amount at once. Repeated quick swallows decrease the time food is held in the mouth and hopefully will speed up Nancy's slow and frequent swallows.
Continue the saliva swallowing exercise.	It is important to maintain skills developed in this exercise.

SIXTH VISIT (2 WEEKS LATER)

Nancy felt she needed more time to practice her therapy and decided to skip 1 week. I explained to her that I understood her desire to be out with her friends instead of having to make the trip to my office and practice therapy. I knew that feeling guilty would not help her progress in therapy but reminded her that therapy would have to be extended if she did not do her exercises regularly. I wanted her to make her own choices, and I reassured her that I would respect the choices she made. Nancy smiled to indicate she understood. I asked her permission to request that her mother help out in a small capacity with the therapy. She agreed.

Home Program	Rationale
Perform the quick swallows with mother observing.	Nancy's mother can help by making sure the exercise is done correctly.
Perform saliva swallows now with a closed mouth with mother observing (three times daily for three swallows each time).	This closed mouth-swallow incorporates a normal breathing and swallowing pattern. Nancy feels safe doing the exercise with saliva. Her mother can remind Nancy to close her mouth when necessary.
Perform the coordinated, closed-mouth swallow with a drop of thinned yogurt if comfortable with the above closed-mouth saliva swallow.	Nancy emphatically requested trying the coordinated closed-mouth swallow with a drop of yogurt at this time. I suggested performing the saliva swallow for 5 days and then attempting the swallow with yogurt.

SEVENTH VISIT (2 WEEKS LATER)

Nancy has made great progress. Closed-mouth saliva swallows and quick swallows with yogurt are now performed comfortably.

Home Program	Rationale
Perform three closed-mouth swallows with the drop of yogurt three times daily. This exercise should be done before each meal or snack and at home away from friends.	Practicing the normal swallow before eating helps Nancy to remember the steps necessary for swallowing correctly.
Eliminate the saliva swallow.	Nancy is now cupping her tongue around the yogurt before swallowing, eliminating the need for this exercise.
Chew three to four small bites of regular textured food slowly. Repeat throughout the meal.	Nancy is ready to begin working with textures.

EIGHTH VISIT (1 WEEK LATER)

Nancy and her mother think they are working well together. Nancy's mother, however, is having to remind her too frequently to do the exercises. I explain to Nancy that it is her responsibility to remember to perform therapy exercises.

Figure 14
Graham cracker exercise to encourage chewing movements.

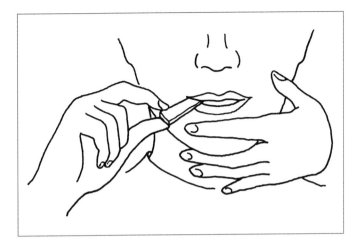

Nancy's progress in the closed-mouth swallow with the drop of yogurt is coming along slowly. She is keeping a chart of her successes and is fairly pleased. She still forgets to chew small bites of food.

Home Program	Rationale
Continue the coordinated yogurt swallow but use a larger amount so that the yogurt covers the entire tip of the teaspoon.	In my office, Nancy tended to place larger amounts of yogurt on her spoon than I had suggested. Instead of making swallowing more difficult (as I had anticipated), the feel of a larger amount of a smooth food makes it easier for her to swallow.
Place a piece of soft but solid cooked potato or carrot between the molars on one side of the mouth. Maintain a *centered* head position while chewing the food. When the food is swallowed, repeat this process on the other side of the mouth. Do this twice on each side of the mouth two to three times daily at the beginning of meals or snacks (Figure 14).	Using a textured food will stimulate and improve lateral tongue movements as well as encourage rotation of the jaw. These movements should help Nancy acquire rotary chewing movements. This is a more advanced version of the graham cracker chewing exercise.
Cut up ¼ of each meal into small bites, place it on a separate plate, and concentrate on chewing movements while eating this portion.	This exercise (done following the above exercise) should help remind Nancy to chew slowly.

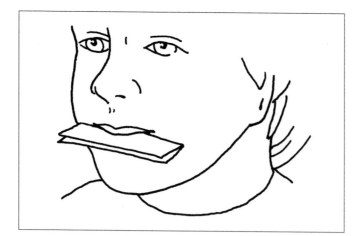

Figure 15
Lip-closure technique using aluminum foil.

Home Program	Rationale
Consult with a speech-language pathologist.	Because Nancy has developed better oral-motor control, her articulation is improving. Working with a speech-language pathologist could help improve her speech skills even more. I had been worried that Nancy would reject the idea of more therapy, so I did not recommend consultation with a speech-language pathologist previously. Mother agreed with me.

NINTH VISIT (2 WEEKS LATER)

Nancy's excessive swallows are less frequent and not quite as noisy (such joy and renewed enthusiasm). She has made an appointment with a speech-language pathologist.

Home Program	Rationale
Place a folded piece of aluminum foil between the *lips*. Record the length of time it can be held before dropping (Figure 15).	The number and loudness of excessive swallows is slowly decreasing. This exercise should also aid in the development of a normal breathing and swallowing pattern. It can be done while Nancy is engaged in other activities at home.
Use applesauce to practice the coordinated swallow.	The coordinated swallow with yogurt is fairly comfortable

Home Program	Rationale
	for Nancy now; therefore, a slightly thicker substance may be used.
Continue the chewing exercise with soft, solid foods, including potatoes, carrots, slightly moist tuna salad, and egg salad, two to three times daily with two bites on each side.	Increasing the variety of textured foods used in the chewing exercise makes therapy more enjoyable.

TENTH VISIT (1 WEEK LATER)

Nancy says she is bored with therapy—not with the exercises themselves, but with "the idea of having to do them." She rarely asks her mother to assist her; therefore, therapy time has decreased. The three of us spent most of the therapy hour discussing and examining Nancy's therapy. At the end of the session, she decided she wanted to stick with it and asked her mother to help her again. The home program for this week remains the same as previous visit's program.

ELEVENTH VISIT (1 WEEK LATER)

Nancy's attitude about therapy has improved because she is seeing significant progress. Her mother and I have observed this progress also. The foil exercise is helping with lip closure and coordinated swallowing. The speech-language pathologist called me. She is very pleased with Nancy's therapy exercises and articulation. We discussed our common goals and agreed that Nancy is doing well.

Home Program	Rationale
Continue the aluminum foil exercise two to three times daily. Increase the time the aluminum foil is held between the lips from 20 seconds to 1 minute (to be done two to three times daily).	Increasing the time this exercise is done will help Nancy develop a normal swallow.
Practice the coordinated swallow with applesauce. (See ninth visit.)	Continued practice will improve coordinated breathing and swallowing with the thickened substance.
Place ¼ of the meal on a separate plate and cut up small pieces. (See eighth visit.)	This routine serves as an ongoing reminder to Nancy to eat small bites slowly.
Continue the chewing exercise. (See eighth visit.)	Integration

TWELFTH VISIT (2 WEEKS LATER)

Nancy is excited about her upcoming driver's license test. She looks forward to more freedom and time with her friends. Her therapy time is even more important to her now because she wishes to progress as quickly as possible to eliminate noisy swallowing and end her therapy.

Home Program	Rationale
Continue the aluminum foil exercise.	Nancy is now able to swallow with a closed mouth for 1–2 minutes, so continuing this exercise will maintain her skills.
Attempt the coordinated swallow with small amounts of a smooth, thoroughly chewed, textured food.	Nancy is comfortable moving on to this step.
Use any textured food for the rotary chewing exercise (see p. 35).	Adding more foods will help Nancy develop rotary chewing skills.

THIRTEENTH VISIT (1 WEEK LATER)

Nancy and her mother report some "family ups and downs" this week; however, some quality therapy time still occurred.

Home Program	Rationale
Practice the aluminum foil exercise twice daily for 5 minutes while reading.	Nancy has developed a good cognitive swallow. She is ready to begin working on a normal, automatic swallow. Focusing her attention on reading instead of the swallow is the first step in this process.
Continue the coordinated swallow exercise with food.	Maintenance

FOURTEENTH VISIT (2 WEEKS LATER)

Nancy reports that she has maintained good cognitive closed-mouth swallows. The automatic swallow has been difficult for her, however. Her mother has seen Nancy chewing too rapidly at dinner. After the usual observation and discussion, we agreed on the home program.

Home Program	Rationale
Practice the aluminum foil exercise two times daily for 5 minutes or more using diversions such as music, television, a book, or homework. Chart the number of minutes the foil is held.	Varying diversions and keeping records of success helps motivate Nancy physically and emotionally.
Eliminate the coordinated swallow with applesauce.	Eliminating this exercise, which has been done successfully, lessens the pressure on Nancy.
Cut up ½ of the dinner into small pieces.	Although Nancy's chewing has improved significantly, she still needs constant reminders to slow her chewing.
Continue the chewing exercise with one to two bites at the beginning, middle, and end of meals and snacks.	Simplifying the exercises will help Nancy complete them. The three periods of placement remind her throughout the meal to chew.

FIFTEENTH VISIT (1 WEEK LATER)

Nancy reports good progress. I observe much less difficulty with the automatic swallow and a quieter swallow! Rotational chewing and articulation have improved significantly.

Home Program	Rationale
Practice the aluminum foil exercise with the coordinated swallow for 5–15 minutes two times a day.	Nancy needs to retain the foil between the lips for as long as possible to develop automatic swallows.
Continue cutting up ½ of dinner.	Maintenance of reminders
Eliminate the chewing exercise.	Nancy's rotational chewing is developing nicely.

SIXTEENTH VISIT (1 WEEK LATER)

Nancy realizes she is doing well and is anxious to complete her therapy. She will continue the therapeutic exercises assigned in the fifteenth visit and return in 2–4 weeks.

SEVENTEENTH VISIT (4 WEEKS LATER)

Nancy passed her driver's license test. She also has an exciting story: "I came into a room full of relatives, stood there for awhile, and when some of them turned around they said, 'Oh, Nancy, you were so quiet we didn't even know you were here.'"

I suggest that Nancy continue her exercises at home and her therapy with the speech-language pathologist, and call me every 2 weeks for 2 months. If progress continues, Nancy's therapy will end. Nancy says she would like to return if she does not continue to progress.

CONCLUSION

Nancy called later and seemed to be doing well. She had finished speech therapy. We said good-bye, although she did ask me to "keep my door open for her just in case." She called again many months later to report that all was well.

I never did understand why Nancy's swallows were louder than those of any other patient I have treated. I am glad that therapy helped her meet *her* goal of quiet swallowing.

Length of intervention: 7 months, 17 visits

The Case of Many Challenges: Severe Brain Damage, Neuromuscular Disorders, and Failure to Thrive

DESCRIPTION AND PRESENTING PROBLEM

Two-year-old Michelle was carried into my office by her mother. At that time I had no idea that I would be working with her for the next 2 years.

Michelle was delivered by cesarean section. She had a low birth weight and severe central nervous system damage. She was microcephalic and hypotonic and had cerebral palsy and failure to thrive. At 8 months, she began having seizures, which are now treated with medication. At 18 months an esophageal fundoplication was performed because Michelle vomited, spit up frequently, coughed, and had chest pains after meals. In this procedure, the fundus of the stomach is wrapped around the esophagus to create a tighter junction. Surgery successfully eliminated the vomiting and chest pains.

Her mother explained that Michelle had feeding problems with both the bottle and spoon. She coughs and cries frequently during feedings and still eats only mashed and blended foods. Michelle's mother seemed very frustrated and eager for help.

Michelle is currently receiving physical therapy at home. I will be in close touch with her primary care physician and physical therapist so that we may coordinate our therapy needs as a team.

FIRST VISIT

The pre-speech, oral-motor feeding evaluation indicated the following dysfunctions.

Dysfunction	Explanation
Bland, droopy facial musculature	Characteristic of persons with hypotonic muscle tone

Dysfunction	Explanation
Absence of head and trunk control; Michelle's head falls backward or forward.	Decreased muscle tone
Open mouth	Muscle tone of the lips and jaws is inadequate to close the mouth, as there is lack of oral-motor control.
Poor (partially reclined) sitting position	Decreased muscle tone
Oral breathing and an open-mouth swallow	Michelle's breathing and swallowing pattern is uncoordinated. (See Glossary, *coordinated breathing and swallowing.*)
Drooling	Poor head and trunk stability and inadequate oral-motor control are major causes of drooling.
Protruding tongue and absence of lateral tongue movements	Because of decreased muscle tone and lack of oral-motor control, Michelle is unable to move her tongue to the sides to pick up food particles and form a bolus. She attempts to swallow by pushing the tongue forward.
Absence of lip closure on the spoon	Because of decreased muscle tone, Michelle is unable to close her lips on the spoon. Food must be scraped off the spoon with her teeth.
Michelle eats only mashed or blended foods.	Michelle rejects all lumpy and textured foods and exhibits oral-tactile hypersensitivity due to central nervous system dysfunction.
Nasal reflux	Food occasionally backs up into the open nasal area because palatal elevation is insufficient.
Liquid intake from a bottle only	Michelle is unable to seal her lips around a cup.
No intelligible sounds	Although Michelle makes noises (cooing), her communication is at the 2-month-old

Dysfunction	Explanation
	level due to developmental delay.
Seizures with eye flutters	Central nervous system dysfunction
Periods of brief withdrawal with blank stares and no movement	These periods do not appear to be due to petit mal seizures.
Lack of environmental awareness. Michelle only seems to be aware of her mother's touch.	Central nervous system dysfunction

Goals

Mother and I agreed on the following treatment goals.

Long-Term Goals

- To improve sitting position
- To improve the texture, quality, and quantity of nutritional intake
- To improve tongue and jaw movements
- To decrease or eliminate drooling
- To acquire the normal, closed-mouth, coordinated swallow and improve the breathing and swallowing pattern

Short-Term Goals

- To stabilize and improve positioning
- To eliminate nasal reflux and coughing
- To improve the spoon technique mother uses at home
- To improve lip closure
- To decrease or eliminate tongue protrusion

INTERVENTION

Mother uses several feeding techniques at home that are uncomfortable and time-consuming. I need to work with her on improving and adapting these techniques.

SECOND VISIT (1 WEEK LATER)

Mother entered my office eager to begin the therapeutic process. I explained to her that at each visit I would observe her feeding Michelle snack foods that she would bring to each visit. Then, I would feed Michelle with other foods of varying textures. We would then discuss and practice the techniques used in the home program. Michelle's mother was intelligent and loving and wished to be completely involved in her daughter's therapy.

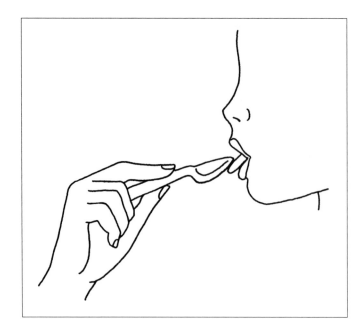

Figure 16
Pressure with a spoon on the tongue to decrease tongue thrust.

Home Program	Rationale
Continue using a tumble-form chair. Use a pillow or wedge of uncovered foam behind the back and head to improve stability and maintain a more upright position.	Michelle needs to be slightly more upright to eat. These changes will make Michelle more comfortable, offer stability, prevent extension of the head, and decrease coughing. The foam wedge is washable and left uncovered to prevent slippage.
Replace the coated teaspoon currently used with an uncoated, shallow spoon.	Michelle needs increased tactile stimulation within her mouth in preparation for accepting textured foods. An uncoated teaspoon offers more tactile input. The spoon needs to be shallow so that Michelle's lips can close down on the food.
Slide a spoon on the tongue over the lower lip at a 45-degree angle with a light but firm touch. Rest the *bowl* of the spoon flat on top of the tongue for 1–2 seconds, two to four times during each meal (Figure 16).	Placing the bowl of the spoon correctly into Michelle's mouth is the first step in using spoon feeding to develop lip closure and decrease tongue protrusion. It also offers tactile input and reduces teeth scraping.

Figure 17
Head and jaw control with the caregiver in a sitting position facing the patient.

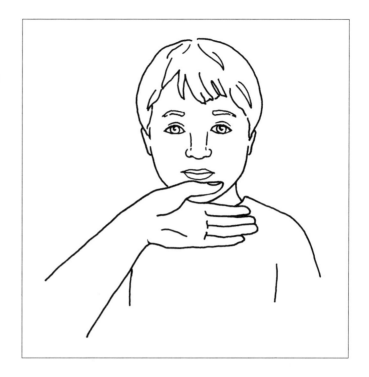

Home Program	Rationale
Pressure with the spoon on the tongue decreases tongue thrust.	I find it more efficient to place the index finger on top of the spoon handle as it helps maintain the angle and keep the bowl of the spoon flat.

THIRD VISIT (2 WEEKS LATER)

Michelle and her mother did very well and are ready for more exercises. Conversation is helping us establish a good rapport.

Home Program	Rationale
Practice positioning at times other than meals. From a seated position, place the back of the hand against Michelle's chest with the thumb under the lower lip to assist in head control. Rest the elbow on a thick towel on the tray for support and comfort (Figure 17). Repeat this position throughout the day.	This positioning technique provides additional sensory input and support for Michelle's head, which frequently flops forward onto her chest or backward. The position of the thumb may also assist in lip closure.

Home Program	Rationale
Fold small amounts of medium-size graham cracker pieces into *each* spoonful of Michelle's mashed food. Prepare these pieces before the meal.	Increasing the texture of mashed and strained foods with graham cracker pieces is healthy and tasty. It begins the process of introducing new oral sensations. Because Michelle demonstrates munching movement, she is able to handle the added texture.

FOURTH VISIT (1 WEEK LATER)

Michelle and her mother consulted with a nutritionist this week. I requested a copy of the report and a consultation with the nutritionist myself so I can incorporate some of the suggested foods into Michelle's therapy. It is also important for the nutritionist to understand Michelle's therapeutic needs.

Home Program	Rationale
Thicken strained foods to the consistency of runny oatmeal using finely crushed graham cracker. Fold medium-size pieces into *each* spoonful. Take tiny bites.	Because Michelle is not rejecting the additional texture and appears to be enjoying the food, the amount of texture can be increased. Mother is reminded to be especially aware of head positioning to reduce or eliminate nasal reflux.
Continue spoon placement as described in the second visit. Hold the spoon on the tongue for 3–4 seconds. Withdraw the spoon in a slightly downward movement over the bottom lip.	Michelle is accepting the spoon placement without discomfort so more time may be added to the exercise. This spoon technique assists in diminishing tongue protrusion while facilitating lip closure.
Use a pillow or foam wedge to keep the hips back in the tumble-form chair. Continue with the wedge for head and neck support.	Michelle's knees and hips require increased flexion to maintain a straighter back.
Continue the positioning exercise described in the third visit.	This position helps maintain body and head stabilization.

FIFTH VISIT (1 WEEK LATER)

I think that Michelle's mother and I have established our comfort zone as we talk to and about Michelle, mother's problems, and life in general. We review techniques so mother and Michelle are as comfortable as possible.

Home Program	Rationale
Continue the technique of spoon placement.	Maintenance for continuing acceptance.
Brush teeth once or twice daily.	Brushing with a soft toothbrush provides tactile stimulation within the mouth, as well as improving dental and gum hygiene.
Continue feeding food with added texture as described in the fourth visit.	This texture provides tactile stimulation in preparation for textured table foods.
Use the position described in the fourth visit on and off throughout the meal as accepted.	Because Michelle accepts this positioning at other times, we may now use it at meals.

SIXTH VISIT (1 WEEK LATER)

Michelle is accepting therapy well but her mother thinks we need to move a little slower. I accept mother's judgment and appreciate her input. I talk with Michelle's physical therapist, who is working on Michelle's overall muscle tone and control.

Home Program	Rationale
Continue all exercises assigned in the fifth visit.	Integration
Place additional spoon pressure on top of the tongue.	Michelle needs firm spoon pressure to prevent the tongue from pushing forward and out and to promote lip closure.

SEVENTH VISIT (1 WEEK LATER)

As I expected, mother is ready for additional exercises because she and Michelle are doing well with the previous assignments.

Home Program	Rationale
Perform the lip-shaking exercise two times, twice daily *before*	Because Michelle and mother are comfortable with the

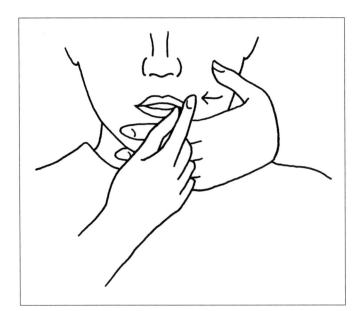

Figure 18
Lip-closure technique using lip shaking.

Home Program	Rationale
meals or snacks. From the standing position, encircle Michelle's neck from the side with the nondominant hand. Rest the index finger under the lower lip with the thumb angled away from the face. Extend the fingers (to prevent squeezing) and cup the chin. Michelle's head will be slightly flexed with the chin "tucked in." Use the right thumb and index finger to gently but firmly shake (or wiggle) the top lip in a downward movement toward the center, beginning first at one corner, moving to the center, and finally to the opposite corner. Wiggle each area three times (Figure 18). Repeat the procedure on the bottom lip using an upward motion.	spoon, it is time to introduce the next step: encouraging increased lip closure on the spoon while enhancing tactile sensation on the lips. This exercise is done in preparation for the spoon-placement exercise. For the standing position described here, caregivers should always bend one leg to protect their back.
Continue the spoon-placement exercise with the index finger on top of the spoon.	Placing the index finger on top of the spoon handle makes it easier and smoother to slide the spoon into Michelle's mouth.

Home Program	Rationale
Observe chair-positioning needs.	Positioning needs are evaluated at each session.
Continue adding texture to food as in the fourth visit.	Integration

EIGHTH VISIT (2 WEEKS LATER)

Mother reports that she is experiencing some minor discomfort. I think that the discomfort may be due to a lack of confidence with the lip-shaking exercise. We review the process (hands-on) and I answer questions and reassure her that both she and Michelle are doing well. Michelle continues to appear comfortable.

Home Program	Rationale
Perform the lip-shaking exercise for two rounds three times a day before meals or snack periods.	Because Michelle's lips demonstrate some closure, we can increase the repetitions of this exercise.
Place a rolled-up hand towel at the nape of Michelle's neck. Maintain hand and finger placement.	Michelle is continuing to move her head excessively in her chair. The towel will assist in improved head control during feeding periods.
Introduce drinking from a cup. Position the hands and fingers as described in the lip-shaking exercise at the seventh visit. Bend over to establish eye contact and observe the mouth.	Michelle is comfortable with the placement of hands on her face for positioning and has begun to develop lip closure, so it is time to introduce drinking from a cup.
Check for some mouth closure while bringing the cup up to the lips and waiting 1–2 seconds for the upper lip to move downward. Teeth will be slightly parted. The head must be slightly flexed as the sip of liquid is simultaneously poured in. Hand placement must remain constant until each swallow is completed. Use a cut-out cup filled to the cut with thinned applesauce or plain, stirred, thin yogurt (Figure 19). One or two sips should be offered occasionally throughout the day.	A thickened liquid is easier for Michelle to swallow than thin liquids. The cut-out cup enables a caregiver to observe the amount of liquid being offered as well as the lip movements for closure.

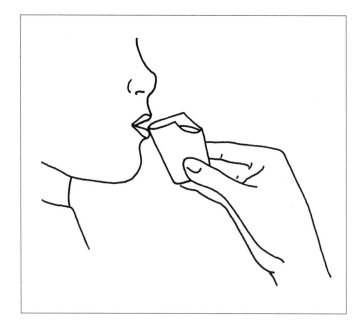

Figure 19
Application of cup pressure on the bottom lip.

NINTH VISIT (2 WEEKS LATER)

Lip closure is improving (although minimally) and Michelle is accepting the cup. No nasal reflux has occurred for 2–3 weeks. Mother is eager to do as much therapy as Michelle will accept.

Home Program	Rationale
Continue the lip-shaking exercise three times a day before meals or snack periods. Follow this exercise with the application of spoon pressure (with a smooth substance such as yogurt).	This sequence of lip-closure techniques follows therapy with practicum. Using snack periods for therapy decreases pressure at mealtimes.
Place medium-size pieces of graham cracker on top of each spoonful of food (instead of folding them into the food).	Increased texture
Practice the chewing exercise with the standing posture used in the lip-shaking and cup-drinking exercises (described in the seventh visit). Place a small piece of graham cracker between the molars on one side of the mouth. When the cracker	This exercise encourages tongue lateralization and jaw rotation. With Michelle's low muscle tone and lack of head, trunk, and body control, only time and effort will tell if chewing skills may be attained.

Figure 20
Graham cracker exercise to encourage chewing movements.

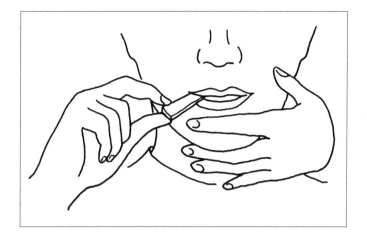

Home Program	Rationale
is melted, chewed, and swallowed, place a similar piece on the other side. Maintain a centered head position (Figure 20). Perform this exercise twice daily (once during a meal and once during a snack).	
After the chewing exercise is completed, offer a few spoons of food with graham crackers on top.	This practicum follows the therapeutic chewing exercise.
Attempt the cup exercise at snack time and occasionally throughout the day.	Snack time is best for practicing exercises.

TENTH VISIT (1 WEEK LATER)

I have been invited to Michelle's school to share my input with school therapists about a new wheelchair for Michelle. I also talk with her physical therapist who tells me he has seen no improvement in muscle tone.

The home program will remain the same as the previous week's program.

ELEVENTH THROUGH FOURTEENTH VISITS (1–2 WEEKS)

The new wheelchair will offer Michelle increased stability and comfort. It should also make feeding a bit easier for her mother by decreasing the need for hands-on positioning.

During these visits, no new problems occur, but lip closure remains minimal. Mother continues with the cup, chewing, and lip-shaking exercises and reports that Michelle appears comfortable and somewhat aware of her environment.

FIFTEENTH VISIT (1 WEEK LATER)

Home Program	Rationale
Continue all exercises (see the ninth visit).	I continue with the same exercises as long as I see some positive, albeit minimal, change.
Increase liquid intake from the cup. Offer three to four sips occasionally throughout the day.	Although lip closure is minimal, cup drinking may be emphasized. Mother and I think that Michelle is ready for this increase.
Eliminate the afternoon bottle.	Michelle's mother wants to eliminate one bottle. Afternoon bottles generally are given up more easily than others.
Continue the chewing exercise.	Michelle accepts the graham cracker between the molars and demonstrates increased munching activity with an occasional lateral movement to the left.
Engage Michelle in activities such as reading stories and playing with textured, colorful, or noisy toys.	Auditory and sensory input will hopefully increase Michelle's awareness of her environment.

SIXTEENTH VISIT (1 MONTH LATER)

I have not seen Michelle for a month due to an illness in her family. The wheelchair has arrived. It seems to suit Michelle well but she still has inadequate head and trunk control. The physical therapist sees no improvement in body tone. We will need to use additional towel and wedge adjustments for positioning in the wheelchair. I give Michelle lots of extra hugs.

Home Program	Rationale
Slide the spoon over the lower lip as pressure is maintained on the tongue for 3 seconds occasionally during the meal (Figure 21). If the lips do not	Increased tactile input and occasional assistance will remind Michelle to close her lips as her tongue protrusion decreases.

Figure 21
Lip-closure technique
using a spoon.

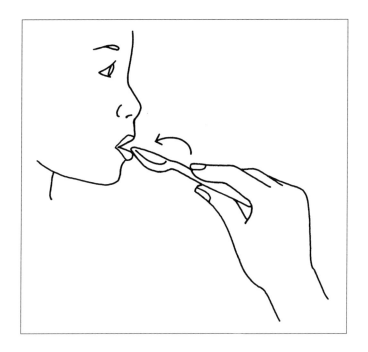

Home Program	Rationale
close at that time, closure may be assisted with fingers.	
Discontinue lip shaking.	Lip-closure exercises with the cup and spoon provide sufficient practice for this skill (a little less work for her mother).
Perform the cup-drinking exercise after the spoon exercise.	Two lip-closure activities, one after the other, provide more input.
Place a rolled-up face towel at the nape of the neck.	Improved positioning in Michelle's new wheelchair (a constant need)
Continue chewing exercises assigned in the ninth visit.	Integration
Continue play activities.	Increased input

SEVENTEENTH VISIT (1 WEEK LATER)

Mother and I see stronger munching movements on the left side and a decrease in drooling and tongue protrusion. Another goal has been met. No change in Michelle's awareness or speech is evident.

Home Program	Rationale
Alternate the graham cracker with soft, solid, cooked pieces of carrot for the chewing exercise (three times daily for one to two bites at the beginning of meals).	Introducing the carrot is a good second step in the gradual process of developing chewing skills. For more information on selection of foods for therapy, see p. 35.
Continue all exercises from the sixteenth visit.	Maintenance and integration

EIGHTEENTH VISIT (2 WEEKS LATER)

Michelle's lateral tongue movements from the side to the middle are somewhat improved and munching is still better only on the left. There is no change in cup-drinking skills and Michelle has not given up her afternoon bottle.

Home Program	Rationale
Continue the chewing exercise with the carrot.	Integration
Attempt to remove the afternoon bottle.	Michelle still wants all of her bottles, but mother wishes to work toward cup drinking.
Continue cup-drinking exercises. Add liquids to foods (per nutritionist's suggestion).	Patients often concentrate on integrating one new skill (e.g., chewing) while regressing or slowing down progress in another area. Michelle is not quite ready to give up any of her daily bottles. When she drinks an increased amount of liquid from the cup, withdrawal of a bottle can begin.

NINETEENTH VISIT (2 WEEKS LATER)

I see a slight improvement in Michelle's ability to move her tongue from one side to the middle. Chewing ability is improving. Michelle demonstrates no interest in play activities but continues to look content.

Home Program	Rationale
Maintain the chewing exercise with the graham cracker on the right molars and the cooked, soft carrot on the left molars	Michelle continues to have difficulty munching on the right side. This exercise gives Michelle increased time to

Home Program	Rationale
(three times daily for two bites on each side at the beginning of meals).	improve her right side chew with graham crackers, which are easier to chew than carrots.
Remember to slightly bend Michelle's head as each tiny sip of liquid is offered from the cup. Begin the exercise with Michelle's mouth in an *almost* closed position. Offer two to five sips occasionally throughout the day. (See the home program for the fourth visit for a complete description of the cup-drinking exercise.)	The cup-drinking posture for caregivers requires time and practice. Coordination is difficult and fatiguing at first.
Continue the spoon exercise.	Continuing integration of skills for lip closure on the spoon

TWENTIETH VISIT (1 MONTH LATER)

Michelle's cup-drinking skill remains about the same, but mother is comfortable and Michelle is content. Chewing skills continue to improve slowly. Her ability to bite down on the left side continues to improve, and tongue protrusion and drooling are greatly diminished.

Home Program	Rationale
Use soft, cooked, solid potato; long cheese puffs; and jicama for the chewing exercise on the left side. Continue to use graham crackers on the right side.	Graham crackers should be used on the right molars because no improvement has been noted on this side. Michelle is biting down and continuing to munch better on her left side, so new foods can be added.
Add crushed bacon bits for added food texture (per mother's request).	Adding textures and flavor may stimulate improved chewing and appetite.
Continue cup drinking (with milk) at snack time and trying to eliminate the afternoon bottle.	Mother is very anxious to eliminate bottle drinking. I always try to comply with a parent's wishes and Michelle is fairly comfortable with the cup now. It is best to encourage cup drinking while slowly eliminating the bottle.

TWENTY-FIRST VISIT (2 WEEKS LATER)

Although mother is showing signs of fatigue, she continues to remain pleased with the changes she sees. The afternoon bottle has been eliminated. As the muscles used for drinking from the bottle and cup are different, it is important to encourage cup drinking as much as possible.

Home Program	Rationale
Continue chewing exercises.	Maintenance
Increase textures of the spoon foods.	Adding carefully selected, soft but textured spoon food encourages increased lateralization of the tongue. For more information on selection of foods for therapy, see p. 35.

Home Program	Rationale
Continue cup drinking at snack time and occasionally throughout the day.	Michelle has accepted the elimination of the afternoon bottle even though she only drinks approximately 2 oz at a time from the cup. The nutritionist is carefully monitoring liquid intake.

TWENTY-SECOND VISIT (2 WEEKS LATER)

We appear to have hit a plateau in Michelle's progress. Michelle appears content but mother is frustrated because she saw no improvement this week. This plateau is not an unusual occurrence, especially during lengthy treatment. Many caregivers and patients experience feelings of anger, sadness, and anxiety after months of daily therapeutic feedings. The successes accomplished seem small in comparison to the work that still needs to be done.

Mother and I spent time discussing her feelings and the progressive steps that had already taken place. I told her that I could not guarantee any particular treatment outcomes but would immediately inform her if I thought we were not making any progress. If this occurred, we could end treatment or I could evaluate Michelle monthly to see if any changes made successful therapy more possible. Whatever would make her mother comfortable was my desire. We talked for an hour and mother decided to continue the exercises assigned in the twenty-first visit.

TWENTY-THIRD VISIT (2 WEEKS LATER)

I talked with the physical therapist, who reported that Michelle was showing few signs, if any, of improvement. Mother understands that developmental delays and poor head and trunk control cause many involuntary movements that make feeding skills difficult to acquire. Controlling the jaw and head has helped, and we are making progress with chewing, spoon feeding, and cup drinking. Cup drinking has finally been accepted.

Home Program	Rationale
Maintain hand position and correct posture for cup drinking and the chewing exercise.	It is important that both mother and Michelle are as comfortable as possible with the necessary exercise positions.
Adjust positions for feeding.	Michelle's head control remains floppy, requiring constant readjustment of mother's fingers. Mother needs to alternate her sitting and standing positions as often as possible for her own comfort.
Use a soft, cooked carrot for the chewing exercise on both sides of the mouth.	Michelle's chewing has improved enough so that more challenging substances can be attempted on the right side also.

TWENTY-FOURTH THROUGH TWENTY-SEVENTH VISITS (ALL 2 WEEKS APART)

The same exercises as for twenty-third visit continued for these four visits.

TWENTY-EIGHTH VISIT (2 WEEKS LATER)

Michelle is showing more interest in food. Lip closure is improving and mother reports practically no drooling. Mother and Michelle are doing a great job. Their perseverance is paying off.

Home Program	Rationale
Perform the lip-shaking exercise from the standing position twice daily (not at mealtimes).	Reinforcing lip closure
Add foods such as scrambled eggs, tuna (with a little mayonnaise), tiny pieces of chicken, and gefilte fish (a soft, solid fish ball; suggested by mother).	Increasing variety of textures
Continue the spoon exercise.	Reinforcing lip closure
Continue cup drinking (see twenty-first visit).	Increasing liquid intake

TWENTY-NINTH VISIT (1 WEEK LATER)

Biting and chewing are still better on the left with slight improvement on the right (especially with the gefilte fish). We reviewed mother's hand position on Michelle's face and chest. Liquid intake is increasing.

Home Program	Rationale
Continue lip shaking (away from meals).	Mother continues to have better head and jaw control from the standing position, and Michelle is just as happy either way.
Cup drinking at meal times.	As cup drinking is accepted by Michelle at snack periods and in the afternoon, we may now introduce it at meal times.

THIRTIETH VISIT (1 WEEK LATER)

I have been working with Michelle and her mother for 1 year now. Mother, Michelle, and I celebrate our successes together with hugs and smiles.

Home Program	Rationale
Continue lip shaking.	Maintenance
Offer the cup immediately after the lip-shaking exercise.	This is an excellent follow-up to the lip shaking to encourage lip closure and increased liquid intake.
Offer one to two bites of a favorite smooth food after the cup.	This is a special therapeutic treat after the cup exercise that encourages lip closure.

THIRTY-FIRST VISIT (2 WEEKS LATER)

Michelle is becoming a bit more aware. She looks around and seems to notice us. She is accepting more and more textured food as well as drinking ½ cup of liquid each time the cup is offered. Lip closure is becoming consistent.

Home Program	Rationale
Discontinue lip-shaking exercise.	Michelle now closes her lips around the cup and on the spoon (once again, a little less work for mother).

Home Program	Rationale
Play activities to stimulate eye-hand coordination for potential finger feeding, reaching for toys, and touching textured objects.	These games take advantage of Michelle's increasing awareness.

THIRTY-SECOND VISIT (1 WEEK LATER)

Michelle is now eating all the soft foods (in tiny pieces) the rest of the family eats (no more mashing). She is beginning to develop rotary chewing movements. Tongue protrusion and drooling have stopped.

Home Program	Rationale
Perform the gum-rubbing exercise two times a day (not at meals), three times each side on the top and bottom gums. Place the tumble-form chair (mother's preference) so it is at shoulder level. Stand on the right side of the chair and encircle Michelle's neck with the left arm, reaching around so that the index finger rests under her lower lip. Angle the thumb away from her face. Extend the fingers to cup the chin for added control. Michelle's head should be slightly flexed with the chin tucked in and the teeth closed. Use the right index finger to rub Michelle's gums firmly back and forth three times, beginning with the top gums. Saliva will be stimulated as the finger is withdrawn and the mouth maintained in the closed position for the swallow.	This exercise is the first step in the acquisition of the normal, closed-mouth, coordinated swallow.
Continue the spoon exercise.	Maintenance
Continue cup drinking. Eliminate the morning bottle.	Michelle is ready for these steps.
Continue offering tactile and auditory stimuli.	Encouraging movement

THIRTY-THIRD VISIT (2 WEEKS LATER)

Mother reports that Michelle has achieved a normal swallow *with* head and jaw control assistance. Her appetite continues improving and liquid consumption is increasing. She shows no change in awareness.

Home Program	Rationale
Continue gum rubbing.	Encouraging the coordinated swallow
Continue spoon and cup exercises.	Maintenance
Observe Michelle's breathing.	Mother is looking to see if breathing is more nasal now that lip closure has improved.
Continue a variety of activities and games.	Encouragement to attain some independent movement and awareness

THIRTY-FOURTH VISIT (2 WEEKS LATER)

Mother has decided to take a well-deserved break. She will call me to discuss Michelle's progress and any problems. I instructed her to stop the gum-rubbing exercise but continue the other exercises. Certain oral therapeutic exercises require close supervision. I talked with the physical therapist, who informed me that therapy is continuing but no change is seen.

THIRTY-FIFTH VISIT (6 MONTHS LATER)

Mother and Michelle return for further assistance. During the break, Michelle's mother kept in touch with me over the phone. She did not ask for a lot of advice but wanted the comfort of knowing I was still there for Michelle and her.

My assessment indicates that very little positive change has occurred but skills have been well maintained. I see no independent eye-hand coordination movements. Michelle and mother have continued their therapy exercises although mother does admit that she has not adhered to a regular schedule as well as before.

Home Program	Rationale
Continue the cup-drinking exercise. Retain the cup on Michelle's lower lip for each sip.	The firm, tactile pressure of the cup on the lower lip encourages lip closure.
Practice the chewing exercise again with textured table foods (not graham crackers).	Michelle does well with soft, solid textures now.

THIRTY-SIXTH VISIT (2 WEEKS LATER)

Mother notices nasal breathing (even during sleep), indicating good lip and jaw closure and perhaps the acquisition of occasional, automatic, normal swallows. Chewing continues to improve with renewal of the exercises. Beginning rotation of the jaw continues to improve on the left side only. The home program maintains the exercises from the last visit.

THIRTY-SEVENTH VISIT (2 WEEKS LATER)

I was invited to Michelle's home to eat dinner with Michelle and her family. She drank clear soup in a cup with head and jaw control. She also adequately chewed soft, textured foods that the rest of the family ate (cut up into small pieces). Head and trunk control were the same. Normal swallows were demonstrated with the assistance of head and jaw control. Michelle and her mother have made significant progress.

    After Michelle went to bed, her mother, father, and I talked. I suggested it was time to stop therapy. Mother and Michelle could manage very nicely by maintaining the exercises. In my opinion, continuing to work on body tone in physical therapy was very important. I told them I would always be there for them. We said good-bye with lots of hugs.

CONCLUSION

A year after Michelle had stopped therapy, her mother brought her to one of my workshops for other therapists and teachers. She told their story and demonstrated all of the techniques we had worked on in therapy for so long. Michelle was now drinking all of her liquids from a cup, chewing soft but textured table foods, and maintaining good lip closure on the spoon and cup. She no longer drooled. She still appeared only slightly aware of her surroundings.

NOTES

- Although I mentioned the role of the primary care physician only once in my account of this case, we had consultations either in person or by phone throughout Michelle's therapy. The cooperation and rapport between the two of us were excellent.
- I have abbreviated this case from 50 to 37 visits. I think that I have covered all of the vital and pertinent facts needed to demonstrate Michelle's problems and treatment.

Length of intervention: 21 months, 50 visits

The Case of the Finger in the Mouth: Prematurity and Developmental Delay

DESCRIPTION AND PRESENTING PROBLEM

Joellen was 21 months old when her mother brought her to my office. She was an adorable blond, blue-eyed child who smiled often. Mother, however, was worried. Joellen regurgitated food and was very difficult to feed. She brought Joellen's medical records, which we read and discussed together. According to these records, Joellen's problems were due to "prematurity and developmental delay." Joellen's smiles and body movements were often meaningless and she made little attempt to communicate. Her mother preferred keeping her at home with her sister rather than enrolling her in a preschool or therapy program. She had only minor physical health problems and took no medications.

FIRST VISIT

Mother fed Joellen her preferred foods: bananas, soaked dry cereal, oatmeal, and strained baby foods.

The pre-speech, oral-motor feeding evaluation indicated the following dysfunctions:

Dysfunction	Explanation
Frequent regurgitation	There appeared to be no medical explanation for the regurgitation.
Sensory defensiveness within the mouth and on the arms and legs. Textured foods were rejected, as well as playing on a carpet or grassy area. She preferred to wear long-sleeved shirts and long pants.	Joellen exhibits sensory defensiveness and rejection due to central nervous system dysfunction stemming from prematurity and developmental delay.

Dysfunction	Explanation
Joellen thrusts her tongue forward and out before swallowing.	This thrusting is a result of abnormal oral-motor control and decreased muscle tone.
Joellen throws her head back to swallow.	Because she has inadequate oral-motor control, Joellen throws her head back to aid in swallowing.
Limited oral intake and nutrition	Because of oral-tactile defensiveness and abnormal oral-motor control, Joellen is a picky eater.
All foods Joellen ate had to be warm and wet and mashed or strained.	Some hypersensitive persons prefer a warm sensation in their mouths. It is easier to swallow strained foods than textured when tongue and jaw movements are abnormal.
Limited tongue and jaw movements. Joellen did not move her tongue and jaw muscles to manipulate food within her mouth. She only swallowed when the food was placed in the back of her mouth. Mother would either drop food into Joellen's mouth or manually close her lips for her.	Abnormal oral-motor control with decreased muscle tone.
Rejection of any liquid from a cup and limited intake from the bottle.	Joellen is unable to close her lips on a spoon or cup because of decreased muscle tone and poor oral-motor control. Even sucking on a bottle is difficult.
Left index finger is always positioned in the mouth during eating.	I did not know why Joellen did this at this time. Her mother did not think it was done to push food out of her mouth or cause regurgitation. It certainly did cause difficulties in feeding.
Open-mouth, oral breathing	Abnormal oral-motor control and decreased muscle tone often result in an open mouth; therefore, Joellen's breathing and swallowing pattern is uncoordinated.

Dysfunction	Explanation
Little awareness or interaction with the environment	This is possibly due to developmental delay.

At the end of the evaluation, Mother and I discussed each problem in detail as well as the normal and abnormal development of feeding skills. I explained that at each visit she and I would feed Joellen. We would then practice the "hands-on" techniques until Mother and Joellen both felt comfortable with them. Finally, we would write up the home program together. We communicated easily. I informed Mother that I would maintain contact with Joellen's primary care physician.

Goals

Joellen's mother and I agreed on the following goals.

Long-Term Goals

- To encourage more normal eating and drinking skills
- To improve the intake of textured foods and liquid
- To use a cup instead of a bottle
- To develop normal breathing and swallowing patterns

Short-Term Goals

- To improve body and head stability during eating
- To decrease or eliminate sensory defensiveness
- To improve tongue and jaw movements
- To encourage lip closure
- To eliminate regurgitation
- To eat a better variety of food textures
- To improve use of the spoon

INTERVENTION

Mother was planning to go to work. I strongly recommended that Joellen be enrolled in a preschool program that would provide social interaction as well as occupational and physical therapy. Mother did not think Joellen was ready.

SECOND VISIT (1 WEEK LATER)

Mother and I both fed Joellen. She was cooperative and comfortable but ate very little even though this visit was arranged to coincide with her lunch time. She also drank very little from her bottle. I made an important observation during this session: Joellen was actually trying to push the food out of her mouth with her finger before she hyperextended her head to swallow. She kept her finger in her mouth throughout the meal.

Home Program	Rationale
Use head control at the end of each feeding period. Place the left arm (as mother is right-handed) across Joellen's back at the nape of her neck, so that the hand rests on the shoulder.	Head control prevents Joellen from hyperextending her head to facilitate the swallow. This position also helps prevent coughing and choking. The position is used intermittently toward the end of the meal so that Joellen's intake will not be decreased by the new technique.
Begin the sensory desensitization process by firmly (but gently) rubbing Joellen's body using up-and-down movements with dry face cloths and towels that have not been placed in the dryer. Legs and arms should be rubbed briskly two to three times daily for 1–2 minutes. The entire body should be rubbed at night, perhaps after a bath.	Firm rubbing decreases sensory defensiveness, in contrast to light touching, which may even increase the problem. The towels need to have a nubby texture. Consistency of the exercise is vital.
Apply firm but gentle pressure halfway back on the tongue with a nonplastic teaspoon holding ½ teaspoon or less of a preferred food. Mother will position herself so that her left hand cups Joellen's chin. The spoon should be at a 45-degree angle as it slides in over the lower lip onto the tongue (Figure 22). This exercise should be performed two to three times during meals or snacks. For more information on lip-closure techniques, see p. 159.	The slight pressure of the uncoated spoon bowl on the tongue provides increased tactile input and encourages lip closure. This exercise will also help decrease tongue thrust. I find it more efficient to place the index finger on top of the spoon handle as it keeps the spoon handle angled and the spoon bowl flat. The preferred food is offered to entice Joellen to eat.

THIRD VISIT (1 WEEK LATER)

Mother arrived smiling. Joellen had not resisted the head control or the towel rubbing. However, she had not been particularly happy with the spoon placement because she now had to work her tongue around the food trying to form a bolus, rather than just letting the food trickle down her throat.

Mother and I talked about her new job and about Joellen (good communication).

Figure 22
Lip-closure technique
using a spoon.

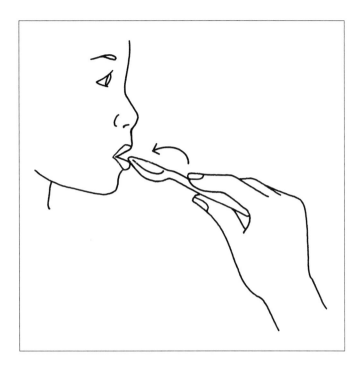

Home Program	Rationale
Continue all three therapeutic exercises assigned in the second visit: head control, tactile desensitization, and the spoon technique.	Continuation is vital for integration.
Sleep in a side position with a firm pillow behind the back, neck, and head.	This position will help Joellen develop additional head flexion. Because Joellen does not hyperextend her body or head when the back of her head is touched, the pillow can be positioned so that her head is slightly flexed. It is hoped that Joellen will swallow her saliva with a closed mouth in this position. This position may also help eliminate regurgitation. Tucking the chin in and flexing the head appears to help form a more cohesive bolus of saliva, which then slowly enters the pharynx.

FOURTH VISIT (1 WEEK LATER)

Mother reports that Joellen continues to comfortably accept the towel rubbing. She occasionally accepts the tactile input of the spoon on her tongue. The sleeping position has presented no problems. Joellen continues to place her finger in her mouth and mother continues to remove it during feedings.

Home Program	Rationale
Continue using the spoon technique, increasing repetitions to three times each feeding period for three bites at the beginning, middle, and end of meals.	It is time to increase therapy periods.
Continue sensory desensitization (towel rubbing).	Continuation for improved integration
Use head control at all meals and at night with the pillow.	Maintenance

FIFTH VISIT (2 WEEKS LATER)

Mother reports absolutely no regurgitation this past week! As I expected, correct head positioning apparently made the difference. She also happily states that she dressed Joellen in short-sleeved shirts and short pants with no protest from Joellen. Two short-term goals have been met. Joellen is also accepting the spoon more.

Home Program	Rationale
Reduce frequency of towel rubbing sessions to once a day.	Maintenance of sensory input for a little longer
Continue head control during sleeping and feeding.	Maintenance of head positioning to prevent regurgitation
Attempt the spoon technique more frequently throughout the meal.	Because Joellen is happily accepting more of the spoon pressure, this exercise can be done more often.

SIXTH VISIT (2 WEEKS LATER)

Because Joellen seems comfortable with the therapy activities tried so far, it is time to begin working on the "finger in the mouth" problem. Now that she is accepting the spoon pressure, I believe that increasing tactile input with textured foods may substitute for the finger. I am eager to increase Joellen's liquid intake; however, I think it is too soon to offer another new therapeutic exercise such as cup drinking.

Mother talks more and more about her job and family life. I think that we have established a comfort zone. Joellen, however, remains inattentive.

Figure 23
Head and jaw control with the caregiver in a sitting position facing the patient.

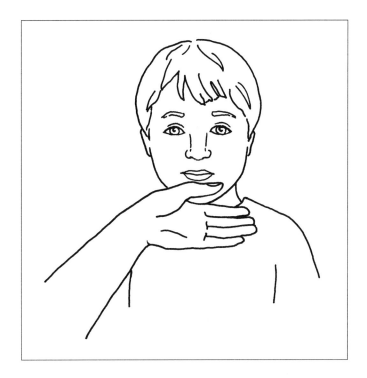

Home Program	Rationale
Increase the texture of foods eaten. Add a minute amount of finely crushed graham crackers to a portion of strained, warm food. Give three bites of the usual warm, strained food for every bite of the warm, slightly thickened, strained food. When this sequence is accepted, decrease the three bites to two bites of the usual food. This may take from a few days to 2 weeks to accomplish.	Joellen will occasionally accept and enjoy some texture within her mouth. Because she is accepting spoon pressure and shows no signs of withdrawal or rejection, I hope this tactile input will prove more substantial than her finger.
Hold the spoon on the tongue for approximately 2 seconds before withdrawing with a downward motion. From a front sitting position, mother will place the back part of her left hand on Joellen's chest and apply light but firm pressure (Figure 23). For more informa-	The light but firm pressure on Joellen's upper chest offers stability while bringing her head slightly downward in flexion. The spoon's downward movement encourages lip closure on the spoon as well as decreased thrusting of the tongue. Mother now has varying posi-

Home Program	Rationale
tion on this technique, see p. 165.	tions from which she can comfortably and therapeutically feed Joellen. This is beneficial to both Joellen and her mother.

SEVENTH VISIT (2 WEEKS LATER)

Joellen's mother has hired a housekeeper named Maria who will accompany her on these visits or come alone with Joellen. Therefore, this visit centered on establishing rapport with Maria while explaining and teaching techniques. Maria is enthusiastic and seems to have a good rapport with Joellen.

The home program remains the same as the sixth visit's program to give Maria and Joellen time to adjust to each other.

EIGHTH VISIT (1 WEEK LATER)

Maria arrived with Joellen. Mother has worked with Maria and Joellen and the transition seems to have gone well. Maria is a bit uncomfortable and shy but is eager to do well. Joellen continues to place her finger in her mouth while eating. She occasionally accepts the two to one ratio of textured food. I encourage conversation with Maria to help her feel more comfortable and relaxed. I continue to consult with Joellen's pediatrician about her therapy, and he is very pleased. He requests an occasional phone call.

Home Program	Rationale
Increase the texture of foods by adding a little more crushed graham crackers as demonstrated. Continue the two to one ratio of strained to textured foods.	Joellen does not appear to resist the degree of texture, just the frequency of the offerings. Therefore, I will not change the ratio. I think Maria also needs more time to adjust.
Eliminate the towel-rubbing exercise.	Joellen is no longer demonstrating sensory defensiveness.
Continue the spoon exercise with slight downward pressure throughout all meals and snacks as often as Joellen will permit.	This should continue to provide the input needed for lip closure and the elimination of tongue thrusting.

NINTH VISIT (2 WEEKS LATER)

Joellen now regularly accepts the additional texture at a two to one ratio (two bites of regular, strained food to one bite of textured food). Maria has stopped warming the strained food and Joellen has not complained. She accepts the spoon pressure

Figure 24
Head and jaw control with the caregiver at the patient's side.

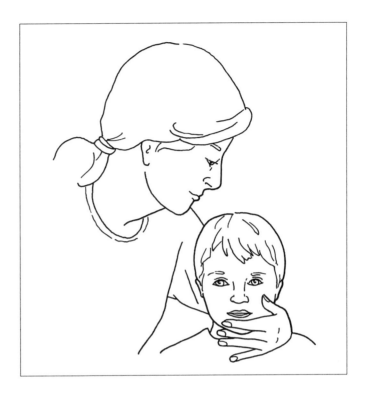

without any problem. Joellen remains fairly passive and does not respond to attempts to interact with her. She only responds to food.

Mother says she added small pieces of dry cereal to Joellen's strained food and that she accepted it. (Mothers frequently know when to make changes.)

Home Program	Rationale
A few pieces of dry cereal or graham crackers will be added into all foods. Maintaining head control is vital.	Joellen has demonstrated that she is ready for added texture. Food intake is increasing.
Place medium-size pieces of graham cracker on top of *each* spoon of slightly thickened, strained food off and on during a meal. Prepare the pieces of cracker before the meal to save time.	This technique should also increase texture acceptance and tactile input. Graham crackers have a crispy texture that melts easily and is therefore safe to use.
Offer a cup containing applesauce thinned with her favorite liquid, milk. Try one sip two to three times per meal. Use head and jaw control from the standing position (Figure 24). For	Joellen demonstrates improved lip tone; therefore, it is time to begin weaning her from the bottle. A thickened liquid is easier to suck and swallow comfortably from a cup and is

Home Program	Rationale
more information on cup-drinking techniques, see p. 171.	less threatening than a thin liquid such as milk, water, or juice. The standing position offers more control for Maria and mother than sitting.
Continue the spoon technique (see the sixth visit for a complete description).	Integration

TENTH VISIT (3 WEEKS LATER)

I thought that Joellen, her mother, and Maria needed more time to become accustomed to the additional therapeutic activities. The dry graham crackers on top of food have been accepted by Joellen. The cup was not accepted—it was probably introduced too early in therapy.

Home Program	Rationale
Thicken food with crushed graham crackers until it is the consistency of oatmeal. Place large pieces of dry graham on top of *each* spoonful.	Because Joellen is beginning to move her tongue, more texture should be added to her food.
Continue the spoon technique.	Maintenance
Add new foods such as spaghetti with meat sauce, mashed potatoes, scrambled eggs, and mashed vegetables.	This will provide additional tastes and soft, mushy textures.
Offer the cup only at snack times.	It is not therapeutic at this time to add more exercises to meal times. However, because the muscles used for drinking from a bottle are not the same as those used on a cup, it is important that we encourage some liquid intake from the cup.

ELEVENTH VISIT (1 WEEK LATER)

Mother tells me Joellen is only placing her finger in her mouth occasionally. The increased tactile input of the spoon and textured food seems to be working! The tongue thrust is rarely seen and the cup is now occasionally accepted for one to two sips. Joellen seems to enjoy her new foods. I encourage mother and Maria to engage Joellen in their conversations each day instead of always talking around her.

Figure 25
Graham cracker exercise
to encourage chewing
movements.

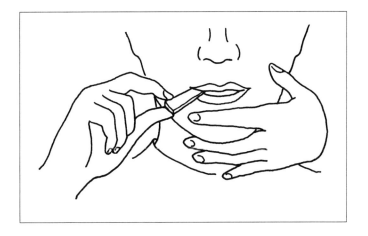

Home Program	Rationale
Practice the chewing exercise with head and jaw control. Place a small piece of graham cracker between the molars on one side of the mouth. Wait until the cracker is melted, chewed, munched, or swallowed. Repeat the procedure on the opposite side of the mouth (Figure 25) for two bites on each side at snack time only. For more information on chewing exercises, see p. 179.	It is time to train Joellen to move her tongue and jaw in beginning lateral and vertical chewing movements. *Head centering* encourages the tongue to move laterally. Performing this exercise at snack time eliminates pressure at meal time.
Continue all exercises outlined in the tenth visit.	Integration

TWELFTH VISIT (1 WEEK LATER)

I requested that both Maria and Joellen's mother come to this session. Because more techniques are being used, it is important that both caregivers continue to follow identical treatment procedures. They report that liquid intake from the cup is only two to three sips a few times per day; therefore, bottle feedings must continue to ensure adequate liquid intake. Joellen is accepting the chewing exercise reluctantly. She demonstrates food likes and dislikes but little improvement in any other form of communication.

Home Program	Rationale
Continue the chewing exercise at snack time.	Because Joellen has not fully accepted this exercise, we

Home Program	Rationale
	must move slowly so that skills can be integrated.
Increase the frequency of cup usage to two to three tiny sips at a time.	Gentle persistence generally pays off.

THIRTEENTH VISIT (2 WEEKS LATER)

Maria, who brings Joellen alone to this visit, tells me that she is now drinking five to six sips of the thickened liquid with the cup (good progress). Joellen's performance in the chewing exercise remains the same. Lip closure is improving and Joellen is placing her finger in her mouth less often.

Home Program	Rationale
Use a favorite food that is *not* eaten at any other time of the day for the chewing exercise.	The enticement of a favorite food encourages chewing movements.
Decrease the amount of thickening of the liquid by half.	Because Joellen's lip closure is improving and sips are taken slowly, it is safe to reduce the amount of thickening.
Offer sips from the cup at the beginning and end of each meal.	Offerings of liquid are no longer annoying to Joellen.
Place small pieces of graham crackers on the high-chair tray for finger feeding.	Maria thinks she sees the potential for Joellen to purposefully move her hands. This exercise will hopefully facilitate eye-hand coordination movements with a safe and tasty food.

FOURTEENTH VISIT (2 WEEKS LATER)

Maria tells me that Joellen appears to search with random hand movements for the pieces of graham cracker on her tray. However, I see no true signs of awareness or purposeful movement. The chewing exercise at snack periods is not progressing very well. Maria and Joellen's mother may be pushing her too hard. I explain that doing too much too soon can actually slow the therapy process. Feeding therapy takes time and patience. It is difficult for caregivers, parents, and patients to move slowly when feeding involves so many hours every day. I offered encouragement and empathy to Joellen's mother and Maria.

Home Program	Rationale
Continue the chewing exercise with a preferred food twice daily at snack time only.	Offering a preferred food at specific therapeutic periods (rather than meal times) makes therapy less stressful.
Include soft but solid pieces of cooked vegetables, such as broccoli and squash, in the menu.	Mother and Maria are anxious to increase the variety of Joellen's food.
Offer the cup of plain milk at snack time (in addition to at the beginning and end of each meal).	Joellen loves milk. With care and tiny sips, she may drink increased amounts of liquid from the cup.
Continue the spoon technique.	Lip-closure exercises need to continue.

FIFTEENTH VISIT (1 WEEK LATER)

Mother and Maria report that Joellen no longer places her finger in her mouth at all. Another goal has been reached! Mother is extremely happy and thinks that she can now turn responsibility for Joellen's visits with me over to Maria. Therefore, she will rarely attend future sessions. Our contact will be through her participation in the home program and telephone calls because she is now working full time. I would prefer that she continue to attend sessions but I understand the situation and am confident that we will continue to progress.

Joellen now appears to be doing well with the chewing exercise and cup drinking. At home, finger-feeding attempts are seen on rare occasions and accompanied by a side-to-side head movement. I suggest placing textured and musical toys on Joellen's table to encourage movement.

The home program is the same as the program assigned at the fourteenth visit. It is best to move slowly so as not to impose excessive input on Joellen.

SIXTEENTH VISIT THROUGH NINETEENTH VISIT (ALL 1 WEEK APART)

In these visits we reviewed home program techniques. Joellen shows no improvement in purposeful hand movements or awareness. Home program remains the same as assigned at the fourteenth visit.

TWENTIETH VISIT (2 WEEKS LATER)

Joellen continues to prefer the bottle to the cup, though she will now take five to six sips of milk from the cup.

Home Program	Rationale
Fill two 4-oz bottles with water and milk and place them in the refrigerator. Record the amount of liquid consumed from these bottles and the cup daily. Add more liquid to foods when possible.	Joellen is now able to drink thinned liquid from a cup and needs only encouragement. Recording will allow us to measure her liquid intake so that we know when it is time to stop bottle feedings.
Practice cup drinking before, during, and after meals, as well as at snack periods.	Continued encouragement
Continue offering the bottle with milk at bedtime.	It is best to maintain a night bottle for the comfort of Joellen and her family.
Perform the chewing exercise twice at the beginning, middle, and end of the meal.	Mother and Maria continue to add soft but solid textured foods to Joellen's diet, such as the broccoli and squash, and Joellen happily accepts them all.

TWENTY-FIRST VISIT (2 WEEKS LATER)

Joellen's mother and Maria attend this session. Mother is anxious and wants to know when therapy will be finished. I listen and then explain again that it is normal for the therapy process to be lengthy and even overwhelming. I reassure her that it is only natural for the family to get upset and wish therapy was over. I then pulled out Joellen's charts so that we could review her progress over the course of therapy. Mother was encouraged by the progress she saw. I asked if she would consider inviting a nutritionist to help with meal planning. She vetoed that suggestion emphatically. I asked if there was anything more I could do. She said, "No, I just need to let it all out and acquire patience and fortitude."

Joellen demonstrates improved vertical and lateral movements of the tongue and some horizontal jaw movements. Tongue thrusting is practically diminished. She is also drinking more from the cup. Many goals are being met.

Home Program	Rationale
Continue exercises from the twentieth visit.	Integration
Increase refrigerated bottles of liquid to two 8-oz bottles.	Joellen is beginning to drink more.
Continue offering the bottle with milk at bedtime. Dilute the bottles of milk given during the day with equal amounts of water. Attempt offering juice.	The nighttime bottle is comforting for Joellen. Increasing the consumption of different types of liquids may hasten her acceptance of cup drinking.

TWENTY-SECOND VISIT (1 WEEK LATER)

Mother sent Joellen's menu for last week, which included tuna, crisped rice cereal, cheese, creamed corn, bacon, peas, pears, peaches, bread, and beef. Mother is much too eager to introduce new foods. The meat and cheese remained stored in Joellen's cheeks and the corn, peas, and tuna had to be mixed with strained foods or they came out whole in bowel movements. The peaches were spit out. Cup drinking is improving.

Home Program	Rationale
Eliminate the foods listed in the menu from last week with the exception of tuna mashed with mayonnaise, bread spread with margarine or butter and cut up into small pieces, *canned* pears, and dry cereal soaked in milk. Only one to two of these new foods should be offered during a period of several days.	New foods should be introduced at a slower pace or Joellen might begin refusing to eat. These foods also need to have a softer consistency. Canned pears have a good texture for chewing. For more information on appropriate food choices, see p. 35.
Mix equal amounts of water and milk for the night bottle. Offer the cup more often during the day. Offer juice occasionally.	These steps are the beginning of the withdrawal of the night bottle.
Continue cup-drinking and chewing exercises.	Integration

TWENTY-THIRD VISIT (1 WEEK LATER)

Maria tells me that Mother is adding strained food to Joellen's textured food, and that Joellen then exhibits tongue thrusting. I will call Mother regarding this problem with the foods. Her liquid consumption (milk and juice) is now 24 ounces daily. The cup is being used more and more. I see no change in Joellen's level of awareness.

The home program remains the same as that assigned for the twenty-second visit.

TWENTY-FOURTH VISIT (1 WEEK LATER)

Mother and I had a lengthy telephone conversation about the addition of strained food to Joellen's meals. She is eager to have Joellen eat increased amounts of food as well as to eat faster. Joellen eats thinner food more quickly. I explained that reducing the textures of Joellen's food had negative results, such as tongue thrusting and the absence of chewing movements. Mother agreed to comply with therapy needs and seemed comfortable with her decision.

Home Program	Rationale
Continue the chewing exercise with soft, solid foods. (See description in the home program for the twentieth visit.)	Integration
Continue offering the night bottle with half milk, half water. Offer a cup of milk just before bedtime.	Joellen does not want to give up her night bottle.

TWENTY-FIFTH VISIT (2 WEEKS LATER)

Joellen now appears to be chewing all the offered textures well. Lateral tongue movements have improved and some jaw rotation movements are beginning to be seen. Overall liquid consumption is now adequate. Joellen continues to demand her night bottle, however. Daytime cup drinking is excellent. The home program will continue as described in the twenty-fourth visit.

TWENTY-SIXTH VISIT (2 WEEKS LATER)

I requested that Joellen's mother come alone to this visit so we could review Joellen's progress again. Many goals have been met, including elimination of regurgitation, tongue thrusting, and the finger placement in the mouth. Food intake, chewing skills, and cup drinking have improved. Mother was pleased to see evidence of Joellen's substantial progress and was glad I had requested her visit so soon again.

I suggested a 1-month "holding" period during which Joellen could fully integrate and enjoy her new skills. At the end of the month, I would begin working on the coordinated breathing and swallowing pattern.

TWENTY-SEVENTH VISIT (1 MONTH LATER)

Maria reported no change in communication awareness. Joellen seemed happy and was eating well.

Home Program	Rationale
Use head and jaw control for the gum-rubbing exercise. Use the index finger to firmly but gently rub the first quadrant of gums on the top, then the second quadrant. Rub three times on each side to create saliva for a swallow. The jaw is held closed gently throughout the exer-	This exercise helps develop a coordinated swallowing and breathing pattern. It was not necessary to rub the bottom gums because sufficient saliva was created by rubbing the top gums.

Home Program	Rationale
cise. Perform this exercise twice daily two times in each section.	
Eliminate the chewing exercise.	Joellen's chewing skills are coming along nicely. It is best to eliminate a successful therapeutic exercise and to concentrate on breathing and swallowing patterns.

TWENTY-EIGHTH VISIT (1 WEEK LATER)

Maria and Joellen did well together this week. Joellen continues with the night bottle of water and milk. I reviewed Maria's hands-on positioning for the gum-rubbing technique.

Home Program	Rationale
Continue the gum-rubbing exercise with head and jaw control.	Integration
Use only water for the night bottle.	This step should keep the weaning process moving along.

TWENTY-NINTH VISIT (1 WEEK LATER)

Joellen remains comfortable with the head and jaw control for the coordinated breathing and saliva swallowing exercise.

Home Program	Rationale
Replace saliva in the gum-rubbing exercise with a tiny drop of liquid for the swallow with head and jaw control (three times daily, two to three sips).	It is time to move from the saliva exercise to more practical applications.

THIRTIETH VISIT (1 WEEK LATER)

Joellen has finally relinquished the last bottle! Lip closure is now excellent on both the cup and spoon and the coordinated swallows are coming along nicely.

Home Program	Rationale
Use a drop of plain yogurt on the spoon instead of the liquid for the coordinated swallow	Joellen is ready to try the coordinated swallow with a smooth food.

Home Program	Rationale
(three times daily, two to three times only).	
Offer small bites of textured foods, including all of the food the family eats.	Jaw rotation continues to improve, so Joellen is ready to try additional foods.

THIRTY-FIRST VISIT (2 WEEKS LATER)

I noticed that Joellen's teeth were not being held tightly closed for the swallow with the drop of yogurt.

Home Program	Rationale
Continue using head and jaw control until a swallow is felt.	Continued reminders will improve Joellen's positioning and swallowing.

THIRTY-SECOND VISIT (2 WEEKS LATER)

Mother and Maria demonstrate their skills in performing therapy techniques. Everyone seems content with Joellen's progress.

Home Program	Rationale
Continue the swallowing exercise.	We are continuing to work toward development of the coordinated swallow.

THIRTY-THIRD VISIT (2 WEEKS LATER)

Mother demonstrated all of the techniques with ease. She thought it was time to stop the therapy visits. She said Maria would continue following the home programs. Because Joellen was eating and drinking well and "only a few problems are left to conquer," she thought it was time to enroll Joellen in a school situation. She would then be able to increase her work hours.

CONCLUSION

Mother called frequently for about 1 year after our last visit. She had been promoted and Joellen was enrolled in a school. Maria continued to be extremely important in their lives—she drove Joellen back and forth to school and cared for her until Mother returned home. Maria stated that Joellen's eating skills remained satisfactory with some "ups and downs."

Length of intervention: 11.5 months, 33 visits

III.

Case Studies: Facility and School Settings

The cases in this section describe the typical differences in care for persons seen in regular weekly or monthly therapy versus those seen on a consulting basis—perhaps for one session or once or twice a year. I strongly believe that all children and adults can be helped in some way even if they have only one therapy session. It is possible to encourage, stimulate, and train staff to consider precautionary measures as well as a few comfortable feeding and vital positioning techniques. Almost all of the staff I have worked with in these situations have been receptive to my suggestions and anxious to help. Teachers, aides, and caregivers who assist with therapeutic feeding guidance deserve much credit for their efforts.

The Case of the Teenage Girl in a Large School Facility

DESCRIPTION AND PRESENTING PROBLEM

I first observed Jeannie in a large classroom with 10 other developmentally disabled teenagers, two teachers, an aide, and a physical therapy assistant who came into the room occasionally to help out. The staff eagerly awaited my arrival because they were anxious to learn how to help Jeannie.

Jeannie is 16 years old and lives at home with her mother. Her medical records indicate that at 18 months she had been "severely shocked by electricity." Soon after, she began to show signs of mental retardation and physical disabilities. She is extremely overweight and sits in a wheelchair all of the time. She communicates with body movements, eye messages, and grunting. The staff appeared to understand and anticipate her every need. Jeannie is very stubborn and occasionally has behavior problems. I was asked to evaluate her positioning needs and feeding problems.

FIRST VISIT (JANUARY)

The pre-speech, oral-motor feeding evaluation indicated the following dysfunctions.

Dysfunction	Explanation
An abnormal, open-mouth swallow with an uncoordinated breathing and swallowing pattern	Inadequate oral-motor control as a result of her neurologic dysfunction
Hyperextension of the head when swallowing	Jeannie throws her head back to aid in swallowing because of abnormal tone and lack of oral-motor control.
Absence of lip closure on the spoon, which causes spillage	Abnormal oral-motor control and muscle tone prevents lip closure on a spoon or cup.

Dysfunction	Explanation
Food is taken into the mouth with a combination of the sucking/suckling tongue thrust pattern. Jeannie is only able to eat small amounts of pureed food.	Neurologic damage causes confusion of movements
Absence of vertical or lateral tongue movements and horizontal jaw movements.	Abnormal oral-motor control with decreased muscle tone
A severe Moro reflex	This primitive reflex causes total body extension. It occurs frequently when she is startled (e.g., when someone opens or closes a door or moves suddenly).
Inadequate wheelchair positioning	Because she has abnormal muscle tone, Jeannie sits in a partially reclined position with her head hyperextended and her legs and hips in extension. Her shoulders are back and purposeful movement with her arms and hands is impossible.

Goals

I knew that I might work with Jeannie only a few times over the period of 1 year. I wanted to set meaningful goals for Jeannie that the staff could realistically work on. I decided on the following goals and then worked with the staff on techniques to fulfill these goals. With their understanding and acceptance of these goals, I observed their follow-through until I was sure that they were comfortable.

Long-Term Goals

- To improve body and head positioning
- To develop the beginning munching skills required for chewing
- To improve the texture of Jeannie's "boring" pureed food
- To develop lip closure on the spoon and cup in order to reduce spillage and improve nutritional intake

Short-Term Goals

- To reposition Jeannie in the wheelchair
- To write a request for a new wheelchair with the physical therapy assistant
- To eliminate the sucking pattern
- To diminish or eliminate tongue thrusting
- To improve lip closure
- To improve the texture of the foods Jeannie eats

INTERVENTION

I explained to the staff that each therapeutic exercise I prescribed had to be consistently performed twice a day. Without consistency, any efforts would be wasted. They accepted this explanation with no hesitation.

Each visit with Jeannie and the staff was about 1 hour and took place in the school room (with the usual and expected interruptions). Because the staff knew my visits might be few in number, they wanted to accomplish as much as possible in this limited time. Each home program exercise was demonstrated in detail.

SECOND VISIT (1 WEEK LATER)

I began by closely observing the teacher and aide responsible for feeding Jeannie her meals. Then I fed Jeannie myself. I discussed Jeannie's wheelchair needs with the staff and the physical therapy assistant. Her current chair was too small but I was told it would have to do for now. Jeannie enjoyed the attention she received during my visit. The home program was coordinated by all of us together.

Home Program	Rationale
Reposition Jeannie in the wheelchair with uncovered foam wedges under the hips, behind the back, and behind the nape of the neck (Figure 26). Place a strap around her waist and in front of her ankles to prevent forward thrusting movements. These are restrictive but *not* tight or uncomfortable. Position a box under Jeannie's feet to encourage stabilization and flexion.	By slowly changing Jeannie's position with these adjustments, she should develop a more flexed posture. Preventing the thrusting movement of Jeannie's body into extension encourages flexion in the hips and pelvis and allows her shoulders and neck to come forward. This relieves tension, encourages relaxation of the upper torso, and improves head control. All of these changes will improve Jeannie's swallow. Hopefully, this position will also diminish or eliminate the Moro reflex.
Add finely crushed graham cracker on top of each spoonful of pureed food. Feed as many spoonfuls as Jeannie will accept during snack and lunch.	The finely crushed cracker adds a new dimension to Jeannie's food: texture. Because this change was safe and not uncomfortable for Jeannie, we decided that the staff could determine how much texture could be added.
Use head and jaw control during feedings. Stand on the	Head and jaw control is necessary for stabilization and cen-

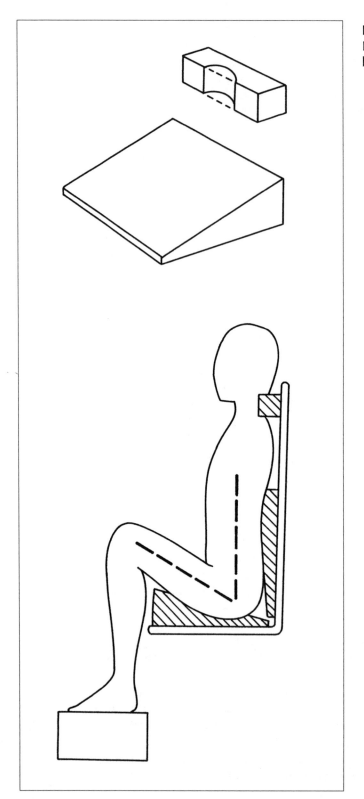

Figure 26
Positioning with foam blocks.

III. Case Studies: Facility and School Settings

Figure 27
Head and jaw control with the caregiver at the patient's side.

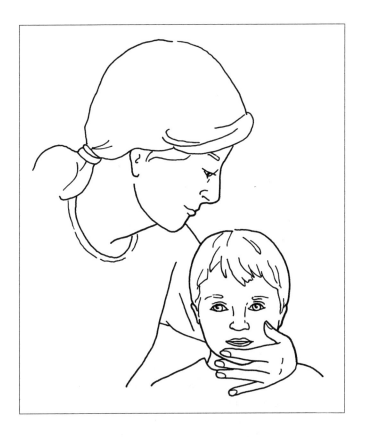

Home Program	Rationale
right side of the wheelchair (if right-handed) and encircle Jeannie's neck with the left arm. Cup her chin with extended fingers. Keep fingers as straight as possible to prevent squeezing motions. Hold the index finger still under the lower lip. Place the third finger just under the chin. Hold the thumb away from the face and eyes. Maintain Jeannie's head in slight flexion with the chin tucked in (Figure 27). Use this position once or twice at the beginning of each meal and snack and once or twice in the middle of the meal.	tering of the head and jaw to prevent hyperextension of the head, assist with lip closure, and diminish tongue-thrusting movements.
Practice the cup-drinking technique with head and jaw con-	The slight pressure of the cup on the lip promotes lip closure.

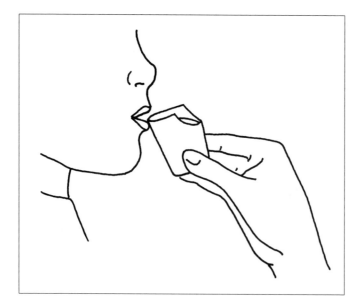

Figure 28
Application of cup pressure on the bottom lip.

Home Program	Rationale
trol. Place a cup of milk on the lower lip with the head slightly flexed. Offer one to three small sips twice a day at the beginning of a meal or snack (Figure 28).	Head and jaw control helps in normal swallowing. Milk is Jeannie's preferred liquid.

THIRD VISIT (1 MONTH LATER)

The staff informs me that the wheelchair positioning adjustments are not working out as well as we had expected. The Moro reflex continues because Jeannie manages to push herself forward into the extended posture. Tongue and jaw movements have improved, however. Jeannie is now demonstrating fewer abnormal tongue movements and beginning munching movements. She continues to enjoy all of the attention and appears comfortable with the new techniques. Because I am uncertain when I will return, I cautiously increase the number of exercises.

Home Program	Rationale
Add more towels and wedges for wheelchair-positioning adjustments. Position an additional small foam wedge cut to fit behind the nape of the neck to allow increased flexion of the head. Place a taller box (or	Because obtaining a new wheelchair for a patient is often a long process, wheelchair readjustments are commonly used in many schools and facilities.

Figure 29
Graham cracker exercise to encourage chewing movements.

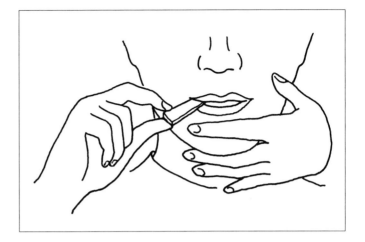

Home Program	Rationale
telephone books) under Jeannie's feet for stabilization and additional flexion of the lower extremities.	
Practice the chewing exercise with graham crackers and long cheese puffs. Use head and jaw control (for a complete description of this technique, see the second visit home program), and place the food between the molars on one side of the mouth. Gently maintain this *centered* head position until the cracker is melted, chewed, or munched and swallowed (Figure 29). Repeat this procedure on the opposite side. Give one to two bites twice daily at the beginning and middle of meals.	Because Jeannie is beginning to demonstrate improved tongue and jaw movements, lateral tongue movements and horizontal jaw movements for chewing can now be emphasized. The graham cracker placement will be used at first, but the crispier cheese puffs add auditory feedback.
Increase the texture of food. Fold medium-size pieces of graham cracker into *each* spoon of food.	Because Jeannie is enjoying the slight change in food texture and is beginning to move her tongue a bit more, more texture may be added. Folding graham cracker into each spoon of food adds texture before the graham cracker has a chance to melt.

The Case of the Teenage Girl in a Large School Facility

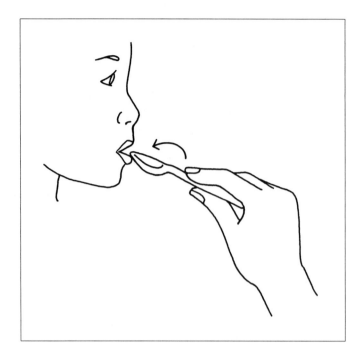

Figure 30
Lip-closure technique using a spoon.

Home Program	Rationale
	For more information on appropriate food selection for therapy, see p. 35.
Slide a spoon in over the lower lip at a 45-degree angle with a light touch. Rest the bowl of the spoon flat on top of the tongue. Apply gentle but firm pressure for 2 seconds. Withdraw the spoon in a slightly downward position while simultaneously offering slight head flexion and jaw closure (Figure 30). Maintain head and jaw control (for head flexion) throughout the exercise.	This exercise encourages lip closure and helps diminish tongue thrusting.
Continue cup drinking with head and jaw control for at least one to three sips. Thicken the milk slightly with applesauce.	It is easier for Jeannie to sip a slightly thickened liquid. Thickened liquid is more controllable and generally easier to swallow than a thin liquid as it moves more slowly into the pharynx.

FOURTH VISIT (MARCH)

Jeannie's positioning has improved significantly. The Moro reflex is practically diminished. Chewing skills and lip closure on the cup and spoon are also improving. We have not heard yet about a new wheelchair. The staff works gently and safely as we progress.

Home Program	Rationale
Continue the chewing exercise with graham crackers; soft, solid, cooked carrot; and cheese puffs. Maintain head and jaw control. Repeat the exercise at the discretion of the staff. Observe Jeannie's chewing skills carefully, including vertical and lateral tongue movements and horizontal jaw movements.	Jeannie is ready to chew a more solid (but soft) substance. The staff will have a jar of cooked carrots on hand to use when this item is not on the school menu.
Enhance the texture of Jeannie's thickened food with larger pieces of graham cracker folded into each bite and dry crushed graham cracker on top of each spoonful of food.	Jeannie is ready for additional texture. If she continues to do well, the staff may request slightly mashed foods instead of the pureed menu. This step is possible because the same staff consistently worked with Jeannie and kept in touch with me by telephone.
Continue the spoon exercise (for a complete description, see the third visit home program). If the wedge at the nape of the neck allows sufficient head flexion, attempt the exercise without head and jaw control.	If the foam wedge offers sufficient head flexion, staff members no longer have to apply their hands to achieve head and jaw control.
Continue the cup-drinking exercise with hands-on head and jaw control.	It is easier to cough, choke, or aspirate, especially with liquid intake, when head positioning is not carefully controlled. Precautionary methods must always be used.

FIFTH VISIT (1 YEAR LATER)

Jeannie continues to improve. She demonstrates adequate tongue movements and beginning signs of jaw rotation. Foods are now mashed with added texture in some meals. The staff is pleased with Jeannie's progress and with their work.

CONCLUSION

Because Jeannie will be leaving this school district, we will send the written therapy programs with her and hope that her new caregivers will be able to continue the program. Jeannie is now comfortable in her wheelchair (she never did receive a new one) and seems happy with her changed diet.

Although Jeannie could have benefited from more therapy, we had been able to make eating safer and easier, positioning more comfortable, and food more interesting.

Length of intervention: 1 year, 4 visits

Acknowledgments
The physical therapy assistant at Jeannie's school was exceedingly helpful, and I am most grateful and appreciative for her cooperation.

I am extremely grateful to the entire staff of the Tulare County Schools in California and especially to Elizabeth Pruitt, the administrator of the severely handicapped programs, who encouraged teachers to schedule a daily "snack module period." This extra period facilitated learning of therapeutic feeding techniques and alleviated a great deal of the pressure that normally falls on the teachers and aides in schools for the developmentally disabled.

Hello, Good-bye
—I Hope
I Helped

The following cases demonstrate that a small amount of guidance, assistance, and care can help persons with feeding disorders tremendously. I often was asked to consult with the staff of schools and adult facilities. I visited facilities for people of all ages and diagnoses. At each visit, I would observe the needs of patients and staff and wish that I could spend at least 1 day in each room or area. I had to do what was possible with my allotted hours, however. I divided my time into segments and worked in each room or area with as many patients as possible. Often I would work with three to four patients per room.

The staff always had charts ready for me and reported additional detailed information as needed. Most of the patients had physical disabilities, mental retardation, developmental delay, or a combination of problems. I would observe a snack or meal period, then feed the patients myself and demonstrate the changes or adaptations that might make feeding easier and safer. I had to consider the limited time caregivers have when making my recommendations. Safe feeding, adequate nutritional intake, correct positioning, and decreasing sensory defensiveness were top priorities. I wrote up detailed therapy programs the day of my visit for the caregivers. This appeared to be a vitally helpful factor to all staffs. While I sought to provide "quick fixes" that were safe, healthy, and comfortable, it would be ideal for these patients to have regular, consistent therapy with an occupational or feeding therapist. If we were lucky, my treatment team would consist of one or more of the following: the teacher or facility director, an occupational therapist, speech pathologist, or therapy assistant or nurse, aide, parent or spouse, and myself.

I hope the following cases from various schools and facilities for the disabled will help readers understand that every person, regardless of age or diagnosis, can be helped in some way. I personally treasure those hundreds of consultation days. (For all of the therapeutic recommendations, see p. 149.)

C.R.
Age: 17 years
Visits: one
Diagnosis: cerebral palsy
Food intake: thickened, pureed food
Problems: seizures, gagging, pneumonia, aspiration
Recommendation: videofluoroscopy (modified barium
    swallow)

A.T.

Age: 1 year

Visits: three (in 3 months)

Diagnosis: developmental delay, poor nutrition

Food intake: small quantities of strained or pureed food

Problems: poor head control, open mouth, hyperextension of the body, lap feeding

Recommendations to mother and staff:

First visit

- Improve positioning in the caregiver's lap, correcting head and trunk control to prevent head and body extension
- Use carrying positions that prevent extension and facilitate flexion
- Add finely crushed graham crackers to food for texture and thickening. For more information on selecting appropriate food textures, see p. 35.

Second visit

- Continue use of carrying and lap positions
- Use a chair for feeding (and play)

Third visit (chair accepted)

- Begin the spoon technique
- Increase food intake
- Consult with a nutritionist

V.T.

Age: 4 years

Visits: two (in 7 months)

Diagnosis: cerebral palsy, spasticity

Food intake: pureed

Problems: absence of chewing skills, hyperextension of the neck

Recommendations:

First visit

- Use head and jaw control during feeding
- Add crushed graham cracker on top of each spoonful of food for texture

Second visit

- Continue head and jaw control
- Add small to medium pieces of graham cracker on top of each spoonful of food for texture
- Begin the chewing exercise when the graham cracker is accepted

J.B.

Age: 4 years

Visits: three (in 1 year)

Diagnosis: developmental delay

Food intake: mashed table food

Problems: munching skill
Recommendations:
First visit
- Use head and jaw control for the chewing exercise
- Fold large-size graham cracker pieces into *each* bite to increase texture
- Add medium-size graham cracker pieces *on top* of each spoonful of food (after the folded-in pieces are accepted)
Second visit
- Use soft, solid foods in the chewing exercise (see p. 35)
Third visit
- Continue exercises (true rotation for chewing was beginning)

S.E.
Age: 17 years
Visits: one
Diagnosis: cerebral palsy, spasticity, quadriplegia
Food intake: cut-up table food
Problems: severe drooling, inadequate nutrition
Recommendations:
- Begin cognitive aluminum foil exercise to diminish drooling
- Practice the automatic aluminum foil exercise while watching television or participating in fine motor activities (after success with cognitive exercise)
- Consult with a nutritionist

D.S.
Age: 10 years
Visits: one
Diagnosis: developmental delay
Food intake: cut-up table food
Problems: lethargy, poor chair positioning, use of hands rather than utensils
Recommendations:
- Consult with a physician about lethargy
- Use a built-up spoon and plate guard
- Give verbal reminders about utensil usage
- Improve chair positioning with a foam wedge placed behind the back to discourage sitting on the spine

M.P.
Age: 26 years
Visits: 2 (in 1 month)
Diagnosis: cerebral palsy, athetosis
Food intake: cut-up table food
Problems: inadequate wheelchair positioning; uncoordinated, open-mouth swallow; poor cup-drinking skills

Recommendations:
First visit
- Request new wheelchair
- Improve sitting position
- Use head and jaw control with cup-drinking technique

Second visit
- Maintain head and jaw control with cup-drinking exercise

F.P.

Age: 24 years
Visits: two (in 4 months)
Diagnosis: cerebral palsy
Food intake: mashed table food
Problems: abnormal open-mouth swallow, excessive head
    flexion, tongue thrust, munching chew only
Recommendations:
First visit
- Use head and jaw control during feeding
- Use spoon technique to control tongue thrust
- Begin chewing exercise with graham cracker

Second visit
- Continue spoon exercise with head and jaw control (F.P. is
  comfortable with both techniques)
- Maintain chewing exercise
- Introduce fun activities requiring F.P. to raise his head (e.g.,
  reaching up to grasp object, wall basketball) during hour
  preceding lunch when possible

H.Z.

Age: 15 years
Visits: one
Diagnosis: cerebral palsy
Food intake: cut-up table food
Problems: H.Z. scoops food independently but takes enor-
    mous bites and has a poor grasp on the spoon.
Recommendations:
- Use a built-up teaspoon and divided plate and place only ¼
  of the meal on the plate.
- Provide hand-over-hand assistance as needed.

R.A.

Age: 17 years
Visits: one
Diagnosis: unknown
Food intake: soft foods
Problems: swollen, bleeding gums
Recommendation: medical referral

D.P.

Age: 4 years

Visits: two (in 1 month)

Diagnosis: developmental delay

Food intake: mashed table food

Problems: Mother feeds D.P. by following him around the house because he refuses to sit in a chair. Munching skill only and a small appetite.

Recommendations to mother and staff:

First visit

Help D.P. become accustomed to sitting in a chair *in between* meal periods. Use television and toys to entertain him while he is in the chair. Extend time in the chair to 10–15 minutes in the first week. D.P. will sit in a chair at meals during the second week. If he refuses to eat, he should be removed from the chair gently and with no sign of distress or anger. He may be returned to the chair off and on all day and offered food. No food is to be offered while he is walking around. Offer him lots of water (not juice) during this learning week. This is a very difficult time but well worth the effort.

Second visit

Because D.P. is now sitting to eat, the chewing exercise with graham crackers can begin.

A.D.

Age: 18 months

Visits: three (in 6 months)

Diagnosis: cerebral palsy, hypotonicity

Food intake: a few bites of strained food

Problems: resists adequate oral intake (previously tube fed), takes only a few sips of liquid (cola) from a cup, poor lip closure, oral-tactile defensiveness

Recommendations to mother and staff:

First visit

- Use sensory stimulation techniques three times a day for 1–2 minutes for 2–3 weeks consistently
- When sensory defensiveness decreases, offer one bite of strained baby food followed by one sip of his preferred liquid (cola)
- Increase to four bites with only one sip of liquid (twice daily, not at meals)

Second visit

A.D. is no longer demonstrating defensiveness. He is accepting increased amounts of strained food without difficulty

- Offer occasional sips of a healthier liquid than cola

- Practice the spoon exercise to improve lip closure
- Practice the chewing exercise with graham crackers

Third visit

A.D. continues to accept increased amounts of strained food but prefers foods fed at home to those at school.

- Maintain spoon and chewing exercises (A.D. does not resist these techniques at all)
- Consider thickening foods with crushed graham cracker in the future

A.B.

Age: 7 years
Visits: one
Diagnosis: tuberous sclerosis
Food intake: cut-up table food
Problems: poor independent scooping of foods
Recommendations:

- Use sticky, lightweight foods on the spoon (e.g., thickened applesauce, whipped mashed potatoes, cottage cheese, whipped cream).
- Staff will place their hands on top of A.B.'s hand with light hand pressure only when it is specifically needed for assistance.

T.S.

Age: 12 years
Visits: one
Diagnosis: cerebral palsy
Food intake: pureed
Problems: hyperextended head in reclining chair; abnormal, open-mouth swallow
Recommendations:

- Modified barium videofluoroscopy to check for silent aspiration
- Correct chair positioning
- Use head and jaw control
- Use spoon technique

IV.

Treatment Techniques: Symptoms, Functional Goals for Treatment, Variations, and Case Examples

I have developed the following techniques after many years of clinical practice. They form the basic structure of my treatment program. Some of the techniques are original and some are based on the research and work of Helen Mueller and A. Jean Ayres. I modify and change these techniques to fit each patient's individual needs based on the sessions with the patient and caregiver.

Techniques for Sensory Desensitization: A Vital First Step

SIGNS AND POSSIBLE SYMPTOMS OF SENSORY DEFENSIVENESS

- Sympathetic nervous system "fight or flight" reaction to touch
- Rejection of touch on any part of the body
- Rejection of oral sensation from food, toys, a spoon, etc.
- Rejection of textured or lumpy foods
- Limited food variation and oral intake
- Preference for long-sleeved clothing to decrease stimuli (e.g., grass, carpeting, toys)
- Abnormal social interaction
- Possible hyperactivity
- Problems with school or learning skills

GOALS OF TREATMENT

A variety of disorders may result in sensory defensiveness. It is vital that all care-givers can touch the patient so that oral therapy can be performed. After the patient accepts touch on the body, head, and mouth, textured foods may be therapeutically introduced slowly while keeping in mind individual developmental needs.

TREATMENT TECHNIQUES

I have found that towel rubbing is always accepted and produces excellent results. Rubbing should be done two to three times daily (never less) for approximately 1–2 minutes. Within a few weeks, positive change may be observed. For more information on the problem of sensory defensiveness, see p. 27. I use the following sequence for towel-rubbing exercises.

Lower body. Rub briskly but gently in an up-and-down pattern with a nubby towel or face cloth that has not been placed in a dryer. During the day, the feet and legs may be rubbed without completely undressing the patient. When lower-body rubbing is accepted, work on the upper body can begin.

Upper body. Rub the arms, fingers, and shoulders briskly but gently in the same up-and-down pattern. The torso is rubbed most easily at bath time.

Full body. Again, bath time is the easiest time to perform this technique.

Head, face, and around the outside of the mouth. These areas are not rubbed until the patient has accepted rubbing everywhere else. Most patients strenuously reject rubbing in this area if it is begun too soon. Use up-and-down movements. During mealtimes, the face and hands may be rubbed or patted dry with the nubby face cloth. For more information on the practical application of sensory desensitization techniques, see the cases beginning on p. 65 and p. 113.

Patients of all ages with sensory defensiveness benefit from exposure to and handling of a wide variety of textures. For hand and body exposure to textures, the following materials may be used.

- Dry, damp, or wet sand. The level of moisture content gives each a different texture as well as varied resistance. For more information on using sand in treatment, see the case beginning on p. 65.
- Clay.
- Boxes filled with multitextured objects (items can also be glued to container lids), such as fine sandpaper, cotton, grass, leaves, silk, corduroy, rice, and beans. Many commercial toys also have varying textures.
- Shaving cream (smooth or textured with sand or rice).
- Hugging games and mouth games. For more information on the practical application of these games in treatment, see the case beginning on p. 65.

Techniques for Head and Jaw Control with Good Body Positioning

This techniques should only be used after sensory defensiveness is greatly reduced or eliminated.

SIGNS AND POSSIBLE SYMPTOMS OF INADEQUATE OR ABSENT HEAD AND JAW CONTROL

- Lack of head and body control
- Difficulty with chewing and swallowing, which frequently limits oral intake
- Difficulty using a spoon and cup
- Coughing, choking, or gagging
- Aspiration
- Uncoordinated breathing and swallowing

GOALS OF TREATMENT

Head and jaw control affects many aspects of feeding and is important in reaching the following goals.

- To gain skills required for adequate oral intake with comfort and safety
- To prevent aspiration of food or liquid into the lungs
- To maintain head and jaw stability and support, encouraging the position needed for improved tongue and jaw movements
- To prevent or control hyperextension or hypoextension when eating, drinking, and swallowing
- To acquire proper positioning of the body, especially the hips, trunk, shoulders, and head
- To decrease or eliminate coughing and choking
- To diminish or extinguish tongue thrusting
- To gain the control required for the normal, coordinated swallow

TREATMENT TECHNIQUES

Head and jaw control techniques should be used intermittently for a few moments until fully accepted. Frequently, it is best to introduce these techniques at times other than meals. A patient is more likely to accept control away from meal times (e.g., playing or watching television). Children respond well to the positive reinforcement of hugs and kisses during these exercises. Before the technique is used during meals, the patient should accept the position for at least 1 minute. Head and jaw control should not feel like a "head lock." It is a gentle but firm control of the tongue and jaw that helps control and diminish tongue thrusting and abnormal head and jaw movements. It also inhibits an exaggerated open-jaw response, which occurs when a patient sees a cup or spoon approaching his or her mouth.

It is also important to never stand in back of a patient, because he or she will frequently look up to see the caregiver's face. The caregiver standing on the side of the patient should always remember to have his or her leg bent (perhaps resting on the rung of a chair) to protect the spine. The following are descriptions of head and jaw control positions for the right-handed caregiver (reverse for left-handed caregivers).

From the side. Correctly position the patient as best as possible to prevent hyperextension or excess flexion of the head and body. Stand beside the chair. Encircle the patient's neck with the left arm so that the extended fingers cup the chin. Establish eye contact with the patient. Keep fingers as straight as possible to prevent squeezing motions. Jaw control should be firm but not too tight and the index finger should remain stationary under (but not touching) the lower lip. The third finger is placed either at the root of the tongue (to inhibit tongue thrust) or on the hyoid bone (just under the tip of the chin). The fourth and little finger are gently placed on the throat so they can feel swallowing motions. The thumb is held away from the face and eyes. The head is only slightly flexed with the chin tucked to create the normal head and neck position for swallowing (Figure 31). For information on the practical application of this technique in treatment, see the cases beginning on p. 65 and p. 91.

From the front. Sit facing the patient to prevent excess head flexion. This position cannot be used for the patient who hyperextends his or her head. Place the back part (dorsal side) of the left hand on the chest directly under the patient's chin. The length of the thumb is positioned under (not on) the lower lip. (Raising the elbow of the caregiver offers increased thumb flexibility.) Rest the left elbow on a tray or on a crossed leg, providing additional support to the arm and hand (Figure 32). For information on the practical application of this technique in treatment, see the cases beginning on p. 91 and p. 113.

For the independent feeder. The patient stabilizes his or her elbows on a table or lap tray and places the fingers of the left hand under the chin with the index finger parallel to and just below the lower lip. The thumb is held parallel to the face and away from the eye. This posture is needed to maintain a normal chin tuck for the comfortable swallow (Figure 33). For information on the practical application of this technique in treatment, see the cases beginning on p. 41 and p. 53.

Figure 31
Head and jaw control
with the caregiver at the
patient's side.

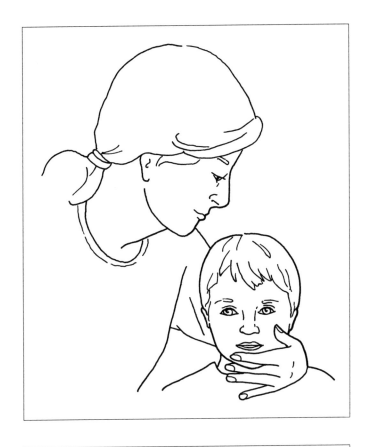

Figure 32
Head and jaw control
with the caregiver in a
sitting position facing the
patient.

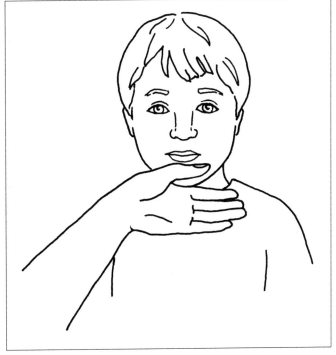

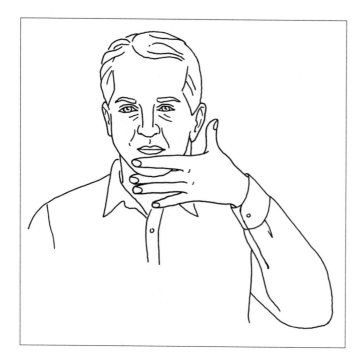

Figure 33
Use of the controlled hand position for independent head and jaw stabilization.

IV. Treatment Techniques

Chin Tuck for Improved Head Control When Swallowing

SIGNS AND POSSIBLE SYMPTOMS OF SWALLOWING PROBLEMS

- Coughing and choking due to excessive head flexion or hyperextension
- Difficulty in accomplishing the swallow due to forward thrusting of the chin
- Difficulty with the chewing process due to forward thrusting of the chin
- Lack of lip and jaw closure

GOALS OF TREATMENT

- To properly align the head, neck, and jaw for more normal chewing and swallowing
- To improve stability and muscle tone

TREATMENT TECHNIQUES

- Elongate the neck with slight flexion of the head (Figure 34).
- Use a standing position for head and jaw control (with a dependent patient). For more information on this technique and its application, see the cases beginning on p. 91 and p. 133.
- Stabilize the elbows on a table or tray while tucking the chin inward and elongating the neck. For more information on this technique and its application, see the cases beginning on p. 41 and p. 53.
- Tuck in the chin (a simple reminder for independent patients). For more information on this technique and its application, see the case beginning on p. 41.

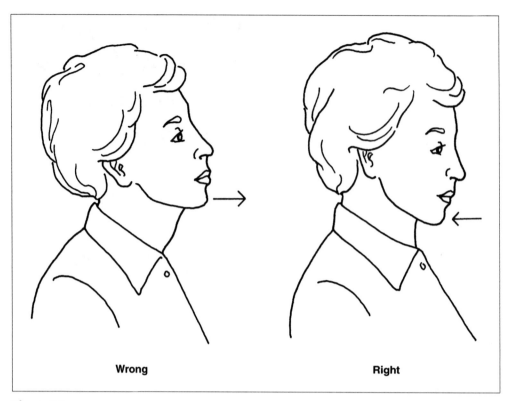

Wrong   **Right**

Figure 34
Examples of correct and incorrect chin-tuck positions.

Lip-Closure Techniques

SIGNS AND POSSIBLE SYMPTOMS OF INADEQUATE LIP CLOSURE

- Drooling
- An open mouth
- Spillage of food and liquid
- Scraping food off the spoon with teeth
- Food and liquid must be "dropped" into the mouth
- Tongue thrust
- Impaired speech

GOALS OF TREATMENT

The mouth must close and the lips seal to accept food or liquid. This prevents drooling and spillage. Improved lip closure helps to decrease the incidence of tongue protrusion.

TREATMENT TECHNIQUES

Lip-Shaking Exercise

The lip-shaking exercise is frequently performed with head and jaw control. The patient or caregiver uses a thumb and index finger to shake or wiggle the top lip firmly but gently in a downward movement toward the center of the lip, beginning first at one corner, moving to the center, and finally to the opposite corner. This exercise makes the lips appear pursed (Figure 35). Each area is wiggled three times. An upward motion is used on the bottom lip three times in each area. It is not uncommon to ask the patient to do only one lip exercise at a time; either the top or the bottom. This exercise needs to be done consistently for two times twice a day. If no change is seen in approximately 3 weeks, the exercise should no longer be used. For more information on this technique and its application, see the cases beginning on p. 53 and p. 91.

Spoon Exercise

The spoon exercise helps develop lip closure and decrease tongue thrusting. A regular, nonplastic spoon provides good tactile input. It should have a fairly shallow

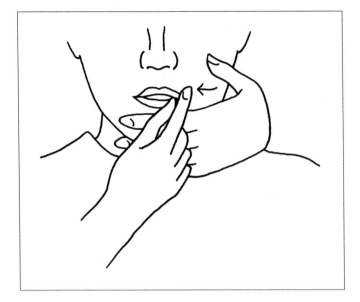

Figure 35
Lip-closure technique using lip shaking.

bowl so that lip closure is not too difficult (Figure 36). Each of the following steps for the spoon exercise may be taught separately.

1. Establish good head and body positioning. Use head and jaw control if needed.
2. Place a medium amount of food on the tip of the spoon.
3. Position the spoon at a 45-degree angle. Carefully slide it in over the lower lip with a light touch. (The caregiver may find it more efficient to place his or her index finger on top of the spoon handle.)
4. Flatten the spoon as it enters the oral area so the *bowl* of the spoon comes to rest flat on top of the tongue.
5. Apply gentle but firm pressure (with the bowl of the spoon) for approximately 2 seconds as the head is flexed slightly.
6. Check for chin tuck. (Steps 5 and 6 are done simultaneously.)
7. Withdraw the spoon slowly in a slightly downward position.
8. Maintain head and jaw control (if used) until the swallow is completed.

For more information on this technique and its application, see the case beginning on p. 53.

Aluminum Foil Exercise

A thin piece of folded aluminum foil is held between the lips (Figure 37). Aluminum foil is the material of choice because it does not stick to the lips (as tissues, paper towels, and plastic wrap do). This exercise can be timed for adults or played as a game with children to see who can hold the foil without letting it drop for the longest period of time. For more information on this technique and its application, see the cases beginning on p. 65 and p. 79.

Figure 36
Lip-closure technique
using a spoon.

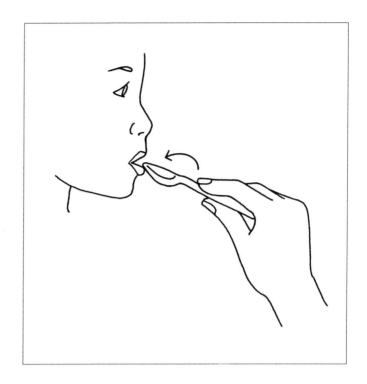

Figure 37
Lip-closure technique
using aluminum foil.

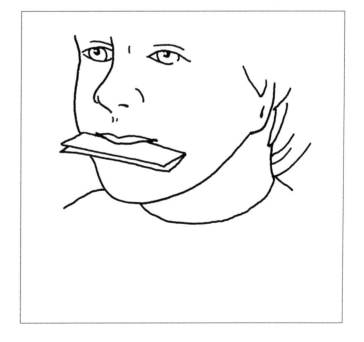

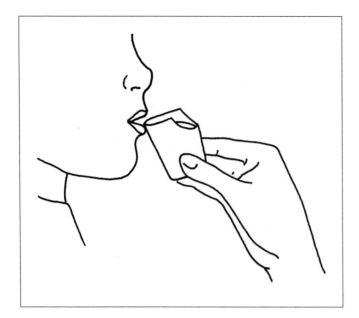

Figure 38
Application of cup pressure on the bottom lip.

Cup Pressure

Maintain slight pressure with the cup on the lower lip (Figure 38) while flexing the head for each consecutive small swallow. For more information on this technique and its application, see the cases beginning on p. 41, p. 91, and p. 133.

Techniques to Decrease or Modify Tongue Thrusting

SIGNS AND POSSIBLE SYMPTOMS OF TONGUE THRUSTING

- Poor body positioning
- Thrusting of foods out of the mouth
- Excess spillage of food from the spoon and liquids from the cup
- Inability to form a bolus with the tongue
- Inadequate tongue mobility
- Poor or absent chewing and drinking skills
- Drooling
- Breathing and swallowing problems

GOALS OF TREATMENT

- To correct abnormal body positioning
- To reduce or eliminate abnormal tongue movements
- To facilitate normal tongue movements for chewing and swallowing
- To encourage lip closure
- To facilitate oral intake
- To improve breathing and swallowing problems

TREATMENT TECHNIQUES

Lip-closure exercises using a spoon can also help decrease tongue thrust (Figure 39). For more information on this technique and its application, see the cases beginning on p. 65, p. 91, p. 133, and p. 159. Cup-drinking techniques can also be used to decrease severe tongue thrusting (Figure 40). For more information on this technique and its application, see p. 175.

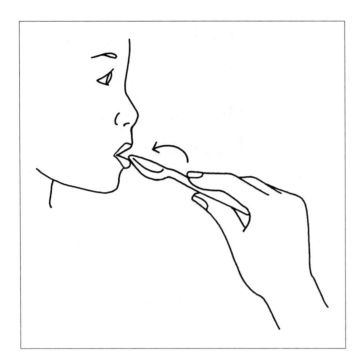

Figure 39
Lip-closure technique
using a spoon.

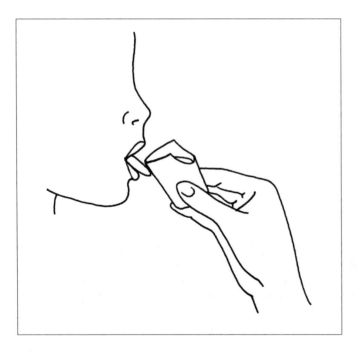

Figure 40
Cup-drinking exercise
with a cut-out cup to de-
crease severe tongue
thrust.

Spoon Techniques for Improved Lip Closure on the Spoon

SIGNS AND POSSIBLE SYMPTOMS OF INADEQUATE LIP CLOSURE

- An open mouth
- Tongue thrusting
- Loss of food out of the mouth
- "Dropping" food into the open mouth
- Scraping food off of the spoon with teeth
- Biting down on the spoon

GOALS OF TREATMENT

- To prevent the bite reflex
- To decrease choking and coughing
- To prevent hyperextension of the head
- To decrease tongue thrusting
- To encourage entrance into a tightly closed mouth
- To encourage lip closure on the spoon
- To improve oral intake
- To make mealtimes safe, comfortable, and clean

TREATMENT TECHNIQUE

For more information on the use of spoon techniques for lip closure (Figure 41), see p. 167 and the cases beginning on p. 53, p. 65, p. 113, p. 133, and p. 159.

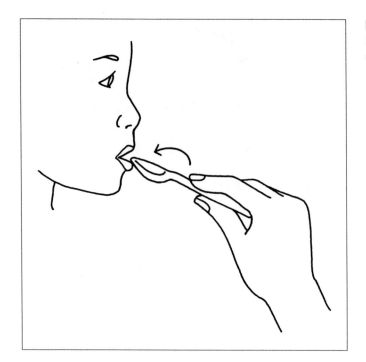

Figure 41
Lip-closure technique
using a spoon.

Spoon Feeding for the Patient with Severe Tongue Thrust

SIGNS AND POSSIBLE SYMPTOMS OF SEVERE TONGUE THRUST

- Tongue thrusting
- Significant jaw extension movements
- An open mouth
- Excessive spillage
- Diminished oral intake of liquid
- Frustration with and rejection of the spoon and cup

GOALS OF TREATMENT

- To eliminate tongue thrust
- To retain the tongue within the mouth
- To encourage lip and jaw closure
- To decrease spillage
- To improve oral intake

TREATMENT TECHNIQUE

1. Position the patient to prevent abnormal extension of the body and facilitate flexion in the knees, hips, trunk, and head.
2. Stand alongside the patient's chair and help him or her assume the chin tuck position.
3. Bend over the patient for eye contact and oral observation.
4. Position the left arm (if right-handed) around the nape of the patient's neck.
5. Place the left hand on the chin of the patient with the index finger under the lower lip and the third finger under the chin at the root of the tongue. Raise the left elbow for increased arm flexibility.
6. Place the *bowl* of the spoon on the protruding tongue and push inward gently.
7. Partially close the jaw with a firm but gentle, slow movement.
8. Firmly but gently close the jaw until it is *almost* completely shut. *Retain this position.*

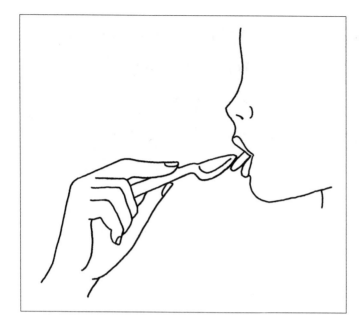

Figure 42
Pressure with a spoon on the tongue to decrease tongue thrust.

9. Slightly flex the head. (The patient's head may need to be leaning slightly against the arm or shoulder to provide leverage.)
10. Withdraw the spoon with a slightly downward movement. (Bilateral lip closure should occur at this point.)
11. Feel the swallow with the third, fourth, or fifth finger.
12. Repeat.

NOTES

Remember to retain hand positioning until each swallow is completed. If the firm grip is lost, the patient's tongue will quickly emerge and the process will have to be started again.

After the first swallow the patient will relax, attempt to close his or her lips for the swallow, and appear to be pleased at his or her accomplishment (Figure 42). For more information on tongue thrusting, see the case beginning on p. 91.

IV. Treatment Techniques

Techniques for Preventing the Tonic Bite Reflex on the Spoon

SIGNS AND POSSIBLE SYMPTOMS OF THE TONIC BITE REFLEX

- Clamping down on the spoon
- Oral hypersensitivity
- Inability to remove food from the spoon
- Inability to remove the spoon from the mouth

GOALS OF TREATMENT

- To break up the abnormal reflex and facilitate a normal response
- To decrease or eliminate oral sensitivity
- To promote adequate food removal from the spoon
- To make the eating process more comfortable for the patient and the caregiver

TREATMENT TECHNIQUE

Sliding a spoon over the lower lip to apply pressure to the tongue can help in the prevention of the tonic bite reflex. For more information on this technique, see p. 159. Correct sitting positioning and gentle but firm use of the spoon are also parts of the process.

If the tonic bite reflex does occur, the spoon can be removed from the patient's mouth by excessively bending the head forward and down. The spoon can then be wiggled gently down and out. This technique may also be used when difficulty occurs due to purposeful behaviors.

Cup-Drinking Techniques

SIGNS AND POSSIBLE SYMPTOMS OF INADEQUATE LIP CLOSURE ON THE CUP

- An open mouth
- Excess spillage
- Abnormal tongue movements
- Diminished oral liquid intake

GOALS OF TREATMENT

Normal drinking from a cup requires that the lips seal completely around the cup edge.

TREATMENT TECHNIQUE

Positioning is important for both the patient and the caregiver while practicing cup-drinking techniques. Many patients with brain damage have abnormal reflexes that inhibit muscle relaxation. In these patients, abnormal hyperextension patterns must be reduced as much as possible before offering the cup to facilitate lip closure. It is also important to correctly position the hypotonic patient. The following steps for the cup-drinking technique offer detailed positioning instructions for the right-handed caregiver. Left-handed caregivers should reverse directions.

1. Stand on the side of the chair, bend over the patient for good eye communication and oral observation, and position your left arm around the nape of the patient's neck.
2. Place your left hand on the chin of the patient with the index finger under the lower lip and the third and fourth fingers extended to partially cup the chin. The thumb is positioned away from the face and the eye and the little finger is gently placed on the throat.
3. Slowly bend the head slightly, gently but firmly tuck the chin in, and almost close the jaw (Figure 43).
4. Maintain this slight head flexion.
5. Pick up a cut-out cup with liquid poured up to the top of the cutout.
6. Maintain an almost closed mouth.
7. Place the cup on the lower lip (Figure 44).

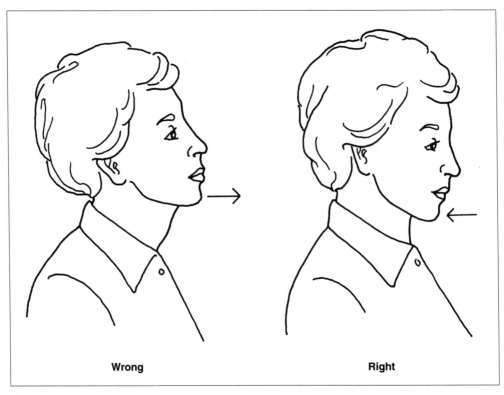

Wrong   **Right**

Figure 43
Examples of correct and incorrect chin-tuck positions.

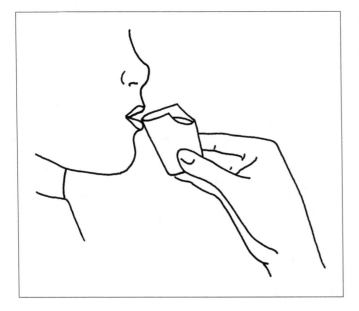

Figure 44
Application of cup pressure on the bottom lip.

8. Pour a small sip of liquid just into the mouth and wait 1–2 seconds for the upper lip to demonstrate a downward movement. (The teeth will be slightly parted.)
9. The swallow may be felt with your fifth finger.
10. Repeat the process. (It may be necessary to pour the next sip before the swallow can be felt.)

Remember to retain the hand positioning until each swallow is completed. In the beginning of this exercise, the normal, closed-mouth swallow may not be attained.

For more information on this technique and its application, see the cases beginning on p. 53, p. 91, and p. 133.

Cup Drinking for the Patient with Severe Tongue Thrust

SIGNS AND POSSIBLE SYMPTOMS OF SEVERE TONGUE THRUSTING WITH CUP DRINKING

- Strong head and jaw extension movements
- An open mouth
- Excessive spillage
- Diminished oral intake of liquid
- Frustration with and rejection of the cup

GOALS OF TREATMENT

For successful cup drinking, the lips need to be closed on the cup and the tongue retained within the mouth.

TREATMENT TECHNIQUE

1. Stand on the side of the chair, bend over the patient for good eye communication and oral observation, and position your left arm (if right-handed) around the nape of the patient's neck.
2. Place your left hand on the chin of the patient with the index finger under the lower lip and the third finger under the chin. The thumb is positioned away from the face and the eye and the fourth finger is gently placed on the throat.
3. Slowly bend the head slightly, gently but firmly tuck the chin in, and almost close the jaw (Figure 45).
4. Maintain this slight head flexion.
5. Pick up a cut-out cup with liquid poured up to the top of the cutout.
6. Maintain an almost closed mouth.
7. Place the flat part of the cut-out cup (not the rim) on the extended tongue and push gently inward (Figure 46).
8. Partially close the jaw with a firm but gentle, slow movement.
9. Wiggle the cup back out to the lips.
10. Almost close the jaw and retain this position firmly but gently.

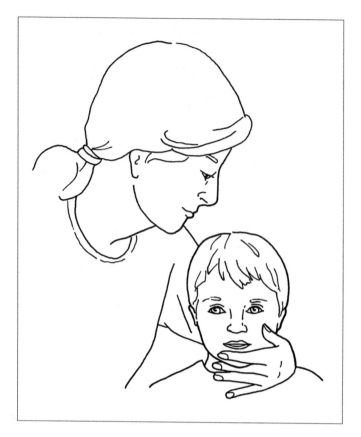

Figure 45
Head and jaw control
with the caregiver at the
patient's side.

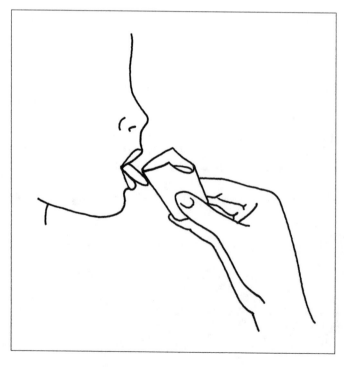

Figure 46
Cup-drinking exercise
with a cut-out cup to de-
crease severe tongue
thrust.

11. Slightly flex the head. (The patient's head may need to lean slightly against your arm or shoulder to provide leverage.)
12. Pour a small sip of liquid just into the mouth and wait 1–2 seconds for the upper lip to demonstrate a downward movement. (The teeth will be slightly parted.)
13. The swallow may be felt with your fourth and fifth fingers.
14. Offer the next small sip *without* removing the cup from the lips.

Remember to retain the hand positioning until each swallow is completed. If you lose your firm grip, the patient's tongue will quickly emerge. In the beginning of this exercise, the normal, closed-mouth swallow may not be attained.

NOTE

In *severe* cases, the swallow may have to be initiated by pressing upward (with the third finger) at the root of the tongue. This should only be done on *rare* occasions.

Techniques for Developing Tongue and Jaw Movements for Chewing

SIGNS AND POSSIBLE SYMPTOMS OF POOR OR ABSENT CHEWING SKILLS

- Absence of normal tongue movements and rotation of the jaw
- Limited intake of textured food
- "Fussy" eater
- Fear of choking or gagging

GOALS OF TREATMENT

The food is moved horizontally, laterally, and in a rotary fashion as it then forms a bolus, which is placed between the tongue and the hard palate in preparation for the swallow. Chewing begins with up-and-down munching movements at approximately 6–7 months of age.

TREATMENT TECHNIQUES

Graham Cracker Exercise

Use head and jaw control and place a small piece of graham cracker between the molars on one side of the mouth. Gently maintain a *centered head* position and wait until the cracker is either melted, chewed, or munched and swallowed (Figure 47). Repeat the procedure on the opposite side of the mouth. This exercise is best done for one to two bites at the beginning of all snacks and meals. When the patient is comfortable with the procedure, it should be repeated in the middle of the meal. It helps to explain to the patient and caregiver that this exercise is a "reminder" to the muscles to chew. The independent patient may perform this exercise without assistance if the head is kept centered. For more information on this technique and its application, see the cases beginning on p. 65, p. 79, p. 91, p. 113, and p. 133.

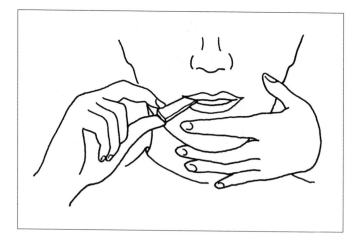

Figure 47
Graham cracker exercise to encourage chewing movements.

Raspberry Seed or Honey Exercise

In this tongue lateralization exercise, the patient or caregiver places a single raspberry seed (from jam) or a dab of honey on the center of the upper lip. The patient then moves his or her tongue upward to capture the seed or honey. If this is successful, the seed needs to be moved 1/16 inch to one side, then 1/16 inch to the other side. This movement continues until the patient is able to touch one or both corners of his or her lip. For more information on this technique and its application, see the cases beginning on p. 53 and p. 65.

Follow the Leader

This exercise can be done if a patient is able to follow instructions. The therapist demonstrates varying tongue movements (e.g., touching one inner cheek, then the other). Speed can be another component of this game.

Techniques to Decrease or Eliminate Drooling

SIGNS AND POSSIBLE SYMPTOMS OF INADEQUATE OR ABSENT CONTROL OF DROOLING

- An open mouth
- Obvious, excessive loss of saliva
- A wet blouse, shirt, apron, or bib
- Wet school papers or desk
- Constant need for a handkerchief, towel, or tissue

GOALS OF TREATMENT

- To remain dry
- To improve lip and jaw closure
- To reduce fear of embarrassment in social situations
- To improve self-esteem

TREATMENT TECHNIQUES

Developing better lip closure is the key to decreasing drooling. Lip-closure exercises, such as the spoon exercise, aluminum foil exercise, and the coordinated closed-mouth swallow, are recommended for this problem. For more information on these techniques and their application, see p. 191 and the cases beginning on p. 53, p. 65, p. 79, p. 91, and p. 159.

Techniques to Decrease Nasal Reflux

In nasal reflux, food and liquid move up, into, and out of the nose instead of being swallowed.

GOALS OF TREATMENT

- To correct the dysfunction
- To encourage the normal pattern of swallowing
- To improve nutrition

TREATMENT TECHNIQUES

Using the chin tuck for improved head control while swallowing to prevent nasal reflux. For more information on this technique, see p. 157. Using thickened food in some cases can also help decrease the occurrence of nasal reflux.

Quick Swallows to Facilitate the Normal Swallow Time

SIGNS AND POSSIBLE SYMPTOMS OF EXCESSIVE BOLUS-FORMING AND SWALLOWING TIME

- Food spreads throughout the mouth
- Excessive tongue and jaw movements before the swallow
- Excessive number of swallows with each sip or bite
- Slow swallows

GOALS OF TREATMENT

A patient may hold food or liquid in his or her mouth for an excessive length of time, perhaps due to an inability to form the bolus in preparation for the swallow. The patient then swallows repeatedly, even with just a minute amount of smooth food. The quick-swallow exercise encourages more normal tongue movements to form the bolus and to swallow more quickly (normally).

TREATMENT TECHNIQUES

The independent feeder can use stirred, plain yogurt (or a similar thin substance). Hold the cup or bowl up to the mouth. Barely touch the yogurt with the teaspoon so that only a drop of yogurt is put on the spoon. When the spoon enters the mouth, attempt to swallow the drop (Figure 48). Repeat this exercise quickly as many times as is comfortable. To vary this exercise, hold a cup up to the lips and take quick sips sequentially. For more information on this technique and its application, see the cases beginning on p. 41 and p. 79.

The dependent feeder is fed by the caregiver sitting in front of the patient. The cup or spoon is held near the patient's mouth and the drop given quickly to the patient.

This exercise needs to be practiced two to three times daily for three to four swallows each time. Approximately 2 weeks of consistent treatment usually produces a positive and productive change.

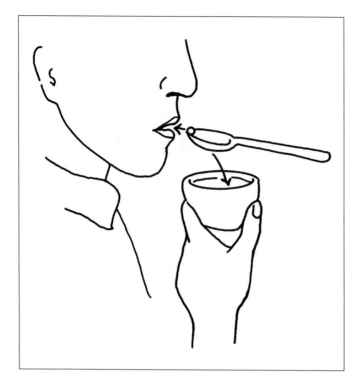

Figure 48
Quick-swallow exercise to facilitate normal swallowing time.

Saliva Swallow Technique for Facilitating the Normal Swallow

SIGNS AND POSSIBLE SYMPTOMS OF INADEQUATE SWALLOWS

- An open-mouth, abnormal swallow
- Hyperextension of the head for the swallow
- Excessively flexed head for the swallow
- Inability to form a bolus for the swallow
- An excessively slow swallow with each bite

GOALS OF TREATMENT

- To encourage the normal, coordinated swallow
- To encourage or improve normal tongue placement for the swallow
- To improve the tongue's ability to form a bolus
- To increase the speed of the swallow

TREATMENT TECHNIQUES

Place the tip of the tongue on the hard palate just behind the upper teeth. Close the lips. The jaw may be closed or slightly open for the swallow, depending on the patient's need at that time in treatment. Head and jaw control may be helpful in some patients. For more information on this technique and its application, see the cases beginning on p. 41, p. 53, and p. 79.

Gum-Rubbing Technique with Head and Jaw Control to Acquire a Normal, Coordinated Swallow

SIGNS AND POSSIBLE SYMPTOMS OF AN ABNORMAL SWALLOW

- An open mouth
- A dry, open mouth
- An abnormal, open-mouth swallow

GOALS OF TREATMENT

This exercise helps in the acquisition of the normal, coordinated swallow.

TREATMENT TECHNIQUE

The caregiver should assume the standing position for head and jaw control. The patient's jaw should be held gently closed throughout the exercise. Insert the index finger to firmly (but gently) rub the first quadrant of gums on the top, followed by the second quadrant on the top. The gums will be rubbed back and forth three times on each side. In most patients, this rubbing creates sufficient saliva to encourage the swallow. If this does not occur, the bottom gums may be stimulated in the same manner. Occasionally, it may be helpful to assist with slight head flexion and the chin tuck position. For more information on this technique and its application, see the case beginning on p. 91.

Techniques for the Development of the Coordinated, Closed-Mouth Swallow

SIGNS AND POSSIBLE SYMPTOMS OF THE UNCOORDINATED, OPEN-MOUTH SWALLOW

- Uncoordinated breathing and swallowing patterns
- Coughing, gagging, or choking
- Aspiration
- Drooling
- Absence of lip closure
- Spillage of food or liquid
- Limited intake of textured food
- Problems with textured, bulky foods

GOALS OF TREATMENT

- To prevent aspiration of food or liquid into the lungs
- To eliminate coughing, gagging, or choking
- To decrease or eliminate drooling
- To decrease spillage
- To encourage more normal breathing and swallowing patterns
- To encourage lip and jaw closure
- To encourage lip closure around the spoon or cup
- To increase oral intake of foods
- To increase ability to eat regular, textured table foods

TREATMENT TECHNIQUES

- Using a spoon (see p. 159)

- Using a minute amount of a smooth food (e.g., plain yogurt, strained food) (see the cases beginning on p. 53, p. 65, p. 79, and p. 133)
- Using a cup (see p. 171)
- Using saliva (see p. 187)
- Using aluminum foil (see the cases beginning on p. 65 and p. 79)
- Gum rubbing (see p. 189)
- Using the automatic swallow (the most difficult and generally the last exercise I offer my patients)

Appendix I
Suggested Reading

Arvedson JC, Rogers BT. Pediatric swallowing and feeding disorders. J Med Speech Lang Pathol 1993;1.

Arvedson JC, Brodsky L (eds). Management of Swallowing Problems. San Diego: Singular Publishing, 1993;327–387.

Ayres AJ. Sensory Integration and the Child. Los Angeles: Western Psychological, 1979.

Bobath B. The Neurodevelopmental Approach to Treatment. In PH Pearson, CE Williams (eds), Physical Therapy Services in Developmental Disabilities. Springfield, IL: Thomas, 1972;144–185.

Bobath B, Bobath K. Motor Development in the Different Types of Cerebral Palsy. London: William Heinemann, 1975.

Bobath K. The Motor Deficit in Patients with Cerebral Palsy. London: William Heinemann, 1974.

Christensen JR. Developmental approach to pediatric neurogenic dysphagia. Dysphagia 1989;3:131–134.

Finnie N. Handling the Young Cerebral Palsied Child at Home. New York: EP Dutton, 1974.

Groher ME. Dysphagia: Diagnosis and Management. Stoneham, MA: Butterworth–Heinemann, 1984.

Klinger JL. Mealtime Manual for People with Disabilities and the Aging. Camden, NJ: Campbell Soup Company with the Institute of Rehabilitation Medicine of New York University Medical Center, 1978.

Lansky V. Feed Me! I'm Yours: A Recipe Book for Mothers. New York: Bantam Books, 1979.

Logemann J. Evaluation and Treatment of Swallowing Disorders. San Diego: College Hill, 1983.

Montague A. Touching. New York: Harper & Row, 1971.

Morris SE. The Normal Acquisition of Oral Feeding Skills: Implications for Assessment and Treatment. New York: Therapeutic Media, 1982.

Morris SE. Program Guidelines for Children with Feeding Problems. Edison, NJ: Childcraft Education, 1972.

Morris SE, Klein MD. Pre-Feeding Skills. Tucson, AZ: Therapy Skill Builders, 1987.

Mueller H. Feeding. In NR Finnie (ed), Handling the Young Cerebral Palsied Child at Home (2nd ed). New York: EP Dutton, 1970;120–132.

Mueller H. Facilitating Feeding and Pre-Speech. In PH Pearson, CE Williams (eds), Physical Therapy Services in the Development Disabilities. Springfield, IL: Thomas, 1972;283–305.

Mueller H. Speech. In NR Finnie (ed), Handling the Young Cerebral Palsied Child at Home (2nd ed). London: William Heinemann, 1974;111–138.

Sheets BV. Anatomy and Physiology of the Speech Mechanism. New York: Bobbs-Merrill, 1973.

Steefel JS. Dysphagia Rehabilitation for Neurologically Impaired Adults. Springfield, IL: Thomas, 1981.

Tuchman DN, Walter RS (eds). Disorders of Feeding and Swallowing in Infants and Children. Pathophysiology, Diagnosis and Treatment. San Diego: Singular Publishing, 1994.

Tuchman DN. Cough, choke, sputter: the evaluation of the child with dysfunctional swallowing. Dysphagia 1989;3:111–116.

Wolf LS, Glass RP. Feeding and Swallowing Disorders in Infancy. Assessment and Management. Tucson, AZ: Therapy Skill Builders, 1992.

Appendix II
Glossary

Abduction	To draw apart (e.g., a separation of the arms or legs).
Abnormal uncoordinated swallow	An open-mouth swallow that causes an abnormal breathing and swallowing pattern.
Absents oneself	The state in which a person demonstrates an apparent unawareness of the environment.
Adduction	To draw together (e.g., bringing the arms or legs together).
Amyotrophic lateral sclerosis (ALS)	Destruction of the myelin sheath of motor neurons along the spinal cord and the brain that results in blocking of nerve impulses. Also known as Lou Gehrig's disease.
Alveolar ridge	The area behind the front teeth on which the tongue tip presses during the swallow.
Asymmetric tonic neck reflex (ATNR)	A reflex in which the arm extends in the direction in which the head turns. It is considered normal in children up to 6 months of age.
Aspiration	The entrance of food, liquid, or a foreign object into the airway. Aspiration pneumonia may result.
Bedside evaluation	A method of data gathering about oral-motor function. Evaluates the history of the problem and use of medications as well as tongue and jaw movements; lip movements on the spoon and cup; normal and abnormal swallows; reflex movements; aspiration; collecting and pocketing of food; tongue thrusting; slow, delayed, or excessive swallows; coughing and choking; a gargling, gravelly, or hoarse voice; excessive drooling; and nasal reflux. Includes a period of discussion that helps in the understanding of the planned treatment.
Beginning chew	The up-and-down action of the jaw known as munching.
Bilabial closure	Closure with both lips to form a seal.

Bolus	A cohesive collection of food formed between the tongue and hard palate before swallowing.
Caregiver	A person devoted to the ongoing care and treatment of a patient.
Cerebral palsy	A central nervous system dysfunction characterized by abnormal muscle movement. The type of abnormal movement is determined by the area of the brain affected (i.e., the cerebral cortex [spasticity], the basal ganglia [athetosis], the cerebellum [ataxia]). Many patients exhibit a combination of these problems because more than one area of the brain is affected.
Chewing	The process of moving food around between the teeth. Movement is controlled by the tongue and jaw through tongue lateralization and elevation as well as vertical, diagonal, and rotational jaw movements. Normal chewing begins developing at 6 months of age and is mastered by 24 months.
Chin tuck	An elongation of the neck with slight flexion of the head and chin.
Cognitive vs. automatic swallows	The cognitive swallow is considered and learned. The automatic swallow is not thought about; it just happens.
Comfort zone	The area of familiarity and comfort that develops through conversation and understanding of feelings of all concerned parties in the therapy process. It provides freedom to share views, needs, and fears without discomfort.
Coordinated breathing and swallowing pattern	The process of alternating nasal breathing with the swallow.
Coordinated swallow	A swallow with the jaw and lips closed as the tongue tip moves forward to press on the alveolar ridge. A bolus of food or liquid then passes down through the pharynx and into the esophagus and stomach. Breathing is nasal.
Cut-out cup	A plastic or Styrofoam cup cut to prevent an adult nose from hitting the cup and to allow a caregiver to see the amount and speed of the liquid being poured into the mouth of the patient.
Dorsum manus	The back side of the hand.
Drooling	An excess of saliva usually seen when teething or learning a new eating skill. Excess drooling may be

related to oral-motor dysfunction or inadequate head, trunk, and jaw control.

Dysautonomia

A familial disorder characterized by abnormal function of the autonomic nervous system. It may result in poor swallowing skills, difficulty breathing, a lack of taste buds and tears, indifference to pain, unstable blood pressure, and motor incoordination.

Esophagus

The hollow, muscular, membranous tube connecting the pharynx to the stomach.

Esophageal fundoplication

A surgical procedure in which the fundus of the stomach is wrapped around the lower end of the esophagus and secured with sutures, creating a tighter junction.

Flexion of the head

Downward positioning of the head.

Floppy movements

An absence of head, trunk, or body control characterized by very loose movements and decreased muscle tone.

Gastroesophageal reflux

Backing up of gastric material into the esophagus.

Gastrostomy tube

A tube surgically placed into the stomach for long-term, nonoral feeding.

Hands-on technique

Demonstration of therapeutic procedures using the therapist's hands on the patient and on the caregiver's hands.

Hard palate

The bony portion of the roof of the mouth.

Head and jaw control

A firm but gentle control of the head, jaw, and tongue that helps diminish abnormal responses while providing support and stability.

Hyoid bone

The structure at the base of the tongue from which the larynx is suspended.

Hyperextension of the head and body

Abnormal thrusting and absence of stability and controlled movement throughout the entire body. May cause an open mouth and drooling.

Hypersensitivity

Intense resistance to touch and sensation.

Hyposensitivity

Very little or no reaction to a touch or sensation.

Hypotonia

Decreased or floppy muscle tone.

Integration

To absorb and learn skills.

Larynx

The musculocartilaginous structure that elevates and closes to protect the trachea so that food and liquid do not penetrate or enter the airway and cause aspiration during the swallow. It is located at the top of the trachea and is also the organ of voice.

Maintenance	To retain, to continue.
Microcephaly	A small head circumference.
Mixed swallows	A combination of normal swallows (closed mouth) and abnormal swallows (open mouth).
Moro reflex	A response to a sudden movement or noise. The body reacts in extension, with abduction of the arms and opening of the hands. This reflex diminishes between 4 and 6 months of age. It is also frequently called the *startle reflex*.
Mouth games	A therapeutic game in which the patient or caregiver lightly bounces a hand or thin scarf on and off the mouth while the patient makes sounds.
Munching	Up-and-down vertical movements of the jaw with no lateral tongue movements. This is the first stage of chewing.
Nasal reflux	The backward flow of food or liquid into the nasopharynx due to insufficient palatal elevation.
Nasogastric tube	A nonoral feeding tube inserted through the nose, pharynx, and esophagus into the stomach. It must be changed every 3–4 days and is usually considered a temporary measure.
Oral-tactile defensiveness	Rejection of touch and texture within the oral area.
Phasic bite	A soft closing and opening movement of the jaw when food or a spoon is placed in the mouth.
Pharynx	The musculomembranous passage between the mouth and the esophagus. The bolus of food passes through it on its way from the mouth to the esophagus and into the stomach.
Positioning	Placement of the body for therapy to break up abnormal reflexes and facilitate normal responses to stimuli.
Pre-speech and feeding muscles	The oral-motor muscles for speech, chewing, and swallowing are the same. Therapeutic feeding therapy may therefore enhance oral skills and speech patterns.
Pursing	The closing of lips as if a purse was being closed with a drawstring.

Quick swallows	A therapeutic exercise with saliva or food to improve slow swallows.
Respiratory deficiency	Uncoordinated sucking, swallowing, and breathing patterns.
Saliva swallows	A therapeutic swallow using saliva only. The tip of the tongue is pressed against the hard palate just behind the front teeth with the lips closed. The teeth may be held slightly open or closed for the swallow.
Sensory defensiveness	An aversion or rejection of touch on one or more parts of the body caused by inadequate integration of sensory information.
Sensory desensitization	Use of towel rubbing, play toys, or textures to reduce sensory defensiveness.
Silent aspiration	Aspiration that occurs with no outward signs of swallowing difficulty (e.g., coughing, gagging). A modified barium videofluoroscopy is required for a thorough evaluation of this problem.
Soft palate (velum)	The posterior fleshy portion of the palate that elevates during the swallow, preventing food and liquid from entering the nasal area.
Sucking	Up-and-down tongue movements with a fair amount of lip closure that creates negative pressure in the oral area. This movement develops at approximately 6–9 months.
Suckling	The early method of sucking (used up to approximately 6 months of age) characterized by extension and retraction of the tongue. Lips are only minimally closed.
Tongue lateralization	Movement of the tongue that propels food to the center of the mouth or to one or both sides of the mouth. This is one step in the rotary chewing process.
Tongue protrusion	Low muscle tone may encourage the tongue to extend out of the mouth.
Tongue thrust	A forceful, abnormal protrusion of the tongue that frequently pushes food out of the mouth.
Tonic bite reflex	Tight closure of the jaw that occurs when a spoon or cup hits the gums or teeth.
Trachea	A cartilaginous tube connecting the larynx to the bronchial tubes—the airway.

Uncoordinated swallow	An open-mouth swallow with oral breathing.
Videofluoroscopy	This modified barium swallow examines the oral, pharyngeal, and cervical esophageal movements and structure during the swallow. It is used to determine the etiology of aspiration.
Volar manus	The palm of the hand.
Walking back on the tongue	The application of pressure with a finger or spoon on the tongue. It is abnormal to accept pressure or touch further than two-thirds of the way back.

Index